SCHIZOPHRENIA AND COMORBID CONDITIONS

Diagnosis and Treatment

CLINICAL

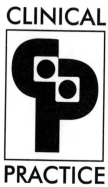

PRACTICE

Judith H. Gold, M.D., F.R.C.P.C.
Elissa P. Benedek, M.D.
Series Editors

SCHIZOPHRENIA AND COMORBID CONDITIONS

Diagnosis and Treatment

Edited by

Michael Y. Hwang, M.D.

Paul C. Bermanzohn, M.D.

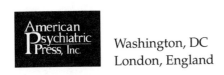

Washington, DC
London, England

Copyright © 2001 American Psychiatric Press, Inc.
ALL RIGHTS RESERVED
Manufactured in the United States of America on acid-free paper
First Edition
04 03 02 01   4 3 2 1

American Psychiatric Press, Inc.
1400 K Street, N.W.
Washington, DC 20005
www.appi.org

Library of Congress Cataloging-in-Publication Data
Schizophrenia and comorbid conditions : diagnosis and treatment / edited
   by Michael Y. Hwang, Paul C. Bermanzohn.—1st ed.
        p. ; cm. — (Clinical practice)
        Includes bibliographical references and index.
        ISBN 0-88048-771-2 (alk. paper)
        1. Schizophrenia. 2. Comorbidity. I. Hwang, Michael Y. II. Bermanzohn,
   Paul C. III. Clinical practice (Unnumbered)
        [DNLM: 1. Schizophrenia—diagnosis. 2. Comorbidity. 3. Schizophrenia—
   therapy. WM 203 S33743 2001]
        RC514 .S33426 2001
        616.89'82—dc21

                                                                    00-058661

British Library Cataloguing in Publication Data
A CIP record is available from the British Library.

Contents

Contributors

Paul C. Bermanzohn, M.D.
Associate Professor of Clinical Psychiatry, Albert Einstein College of Medicine, New York, New York; Medical Director, Queen's Day Center, Hillside Hospital/North Shore–Long Island Jewish Health System, Jamaica, New York

Leslie Citrome, M.D., M.P.H.
Clinical Associate Professor of Psychiatry, New York University, New York, New York; Director, Clinical Research and Evaluation Facility, Nathan S. Kline Institute for Psychiatric Research, Orangeburg, New York

John H. Eastham, Pharm.D.
Clinical Specialist, Department of Pharmacy, Naval Medical Center San Diego, San Diego, California; Clinical Assistant Professor of Pharmacy Practice, Western University of Health Sciences, Pomona, California

John H. Gilmore, M.D.
Associate Professor, Department of Psychiatry, University of North Carolina School of Medicine, Chapel Hill

J. Akiko Gladsjo, Ph.D.
Research Fellow in Geriatric Psychiatry, University of California, San Diego; San Diego VA Medical Center, San Diego, California

Michael Y. Hwang, M.D.
Associate Professor of Psychiatry, Robert Wood Johnson Medical School—UMDNJ, Piscataway, New Jersey; Director of Schizophrenia Research, East Orange VAMC, East Orange, New Jersey

L. Fredrik Jarskog, M.D.
Assistant Professor, Department of Psychiatry, University of North Carolina School of Medicine, Chapel Hill

Dilip V. Jeste, M.D.
Professor of Psychiatry and Neurosciences, University of California, San Diego; San Diego VA Medical Center, San Diego, California

Connie Nickou, Psy.D.
Clinical Instructor, Department of Psychiatry, Yale University, New Haven, Connecticut

Lewis A. Opler, M.D., Ph.D.
Adjunct Professor of Psychiatry, Columbia University College of Physicians and Surgeons, New York, New York; Director of Research Division, New York State Office of Mental Health, New York, New York

Richard J. Pitch, M.D.
Private practice, Melville, New York

Simcha Pollack, Ph.D.
Formerly Biostatistician, Department of Research, Hillside Hospital/North Shore–Long Island Jewish Health System, Jamaica, New York; currently Professor of Statistics, Department of Computer Information Systems and Decision Sciences, St. John's University, Jamaica, New York

Linda Porto, M.S.N., R.N., C.S.
Research Nurse, Department of Research, Hillside Hospital/North Shore–Long Island Jewish Health System, Glen Oaks, New York

Samuel G. Siris, M.D.
Professor of Psychiatry, Albert Einstein College of Medicine, New York, New York; Director, Division of Continuing Psychiatric Services for Schizophrenia and Related Conditions, Hillside Hospital/North Shore–Long Island Jewish Health System, Glen Oaks, New York

Roz Stronger, M.A.
Application Support Specialist, Hillside Hospital/North Shore–Long Island Jewish Health System, Glen Oaks, New York

T. Scott Stroup, M.D., M.P.H.
Assistant Professor, Department of Psychiatry, University of North Carolina School of Medicine, Chapel Hill

Jan Volavka, M.D., Ph.D.
Professor of Psychiatry, New York University, New York, New York; Chief, Clinical Research Division, Nathan S. Kline Institute for Psychiatric Research, Orangeburg, New York

Douglas Ziedonis, M.D., M.P.H.
Associate Professor and Director, Division of Addiction Psychiatry, Robert Wood Johnson Medical School, Piscataway, New Jersey

Introduction
to the Clinical Practice Series

*T*he Clinical Practice Series is dedicated to the support of continuing education and enrichment for the practicing clinician. Books in this series address topics of concern and importance to psychiatrists and other mental health clinicians. Each volume provides up-to-date literature reviews and emphasizes the most recent treatment approaches to psychiatric illnesses. Theoretical and scientific data are applied to clinical situations, and case illustrations are used extensively to increase the relevance of the material for the practitioner.

Each year the series publishes a number of books dealing with all aspects of clinical practice. From time to time some of these publications may be revised and updated. Some books in the series are written by a single clinician widely acknowledged to be an authority on the topic area; other series books are edited volumes in which knowledgeable practitioners contribute chapters in their areas of expertise. Still other series books have their origins in presentations for an American Psychiatric Association Annual Meeting. All contain the newest research and clinical information available on the subjects discussed.

The Clinical Practice Series provides enrichment reading in a compact format specially designed to meet the continuing-education needs of the busy mental health clinician.

Judith H. Gold, C.M., M.D., F.R.C.P.C., F.R.A.N.Z.C.P.
Series Editor

Preface

Michael Y. Hwang, M.D.
Paul C. Bermanzohn, M.D.

*T*he idea for this monograph was born years ago after a symposium at the American Psychiatric Association on comorbid disorders in schizophrenia. The presenters at that symposium, many of whom have authored chapters in this book, agreed that there was a deficiency in clinical guidelines for the management of schizophrenia patients with comorbid conditions. They also agreed that the traditional approach to the diagnosis of psychiatric disorders, which precluded additional diagnoses in the presence of schizophrenia, created many problems. One result of such diagnostic limitations is that there have been few controlled studies to examine patients with these complex, comorbid conditions. Since that time, however, there have been important changes in the approach to diagnosis in schizophrenia. DSM-IV, published in 1994, now permits additional diagnoses on Axis I, such as anxiety disorders, in the presence of schizophrenia. This change in diagnostic practice has been associated with an increase in the number of studies of comorbidity. This expanded interest has led to a greater recognition of comorbidity in schizophrenia patients and of the idea that these patients should be managed based on their individual clinical presentations rather than simply based on their categorical diagnosis.

Two leaders in the field, Herman M. Van Praag and John S. Strauss, have inspired much of our work. Professor Van Praag has long advocated a multitiered diagnostic system that would recognize syndromal as well as categorical diagnosis in psychiatric illness (Van Praag et al. 1990). Dr. John S. Strauss has devoted his career to questioning the simplifications of schizophrenia, the symptoms for which may seem clear or compelling on paper but do not accurately describe clinical phenomena. He has called on psychiatry to honestly look at our patients' experiences (Strauss 1989). The strong convictions of both these teachers have helped to shape our views, especially in questioning the idea that "all schizophrenics are the same."

The primary goal of this monograph is to help practicing clinicians enhance their recognition and improve treatment for this large and difficult-to-treat group of schizophrenia patients. We hope to present currently available information in an organized and useful format and, where possible, to suggest guidelines in patient management.

We have been indeed fortunate in that our authors combine a wealth of clinical and research experience, enabling them to help guide us through these complex clinical phenomena. In Chapter 1, Dr. Bermanzohn and colleagues present an overview of associated psychiatric syndromes, or APS, in schizophrenia, particularly depression, obsessive-compulsive disorder, and panic disorder. They criticize the reductionist view of schizophrenia as a single unitary disorder, a view that leads to ignoring these potentially important syndromes. In Chapter 2, Dr. Siris reviews the extensive literature on depression in schizophrenia and discusses differential diagnosis and treatment approaches in this long-recognized comorbid condition. Drs. Hwang and Pitch and colleagues, in Chapters 3 and 4, present information on schizophrenia with obsessive-compulsive and panic symptoms, respectively, and discuss clinical management of these conditions by means of clinical case vignettes. This is an evolving area in which we expect significant advances in the future. In Chapters 5 and 6, Dr. Gilmore and colleagues discuss medical illness and pregnancy in schizophrenia, focusing on management of these conditions. In Chapter 7, Dr. Gladsjo and associates review cognitive impairment in schizophrenia and discuss assessment and treatment issues. Drs. Citrome and Volavka, in Chapter 8, review aggressive behaviors in schizophrenia and discuss old and new treatment approaches for this challenging group of patients. Finally, Drs. Ziedonis and Nickou extensively review substance abuse in schizophrenia and suggest practical approaches in the assessment and treatment of the "dual-diagnosis" schizophrenia patient.

We hope this collection will enhance clinical care for these often neglected and clinically challenging patients.

References

Strauss JS: Subjective experiences of schizophrenia: toward a new dynamic psychiatry—II. Schizophr Bull 15:179–187, 1989

Van Praag HM, Asnis GM, Kahn RS, et al: Nosological tunnel vision in biological psychiatry. Ann N Y Acad Sci 600:501–510, 1990

Acknowledgments

*T*he editors would like to acknowledge the conceptual inspirations for this monograph from H. Van Praag, M.D., Ph.D., and John Strauss, M.D., who have long advocated for the symptom–based approach in the management of schizophrenic illness. We would also like to acknowledge Lewis A. Opler, M.D., and Eric Hollander, M.D., for their continued support and scientific inspirations. In addition, we are grateful for our families' support.

This work was funded in part by an American Psychiatric Association/National Institute of Mental Health postdoctoral grant (MH-19126) to Dr. Hwang, and a Young Investigators Award from the National Alliance for Research in Schizophrenia and Depression and a staff society grant from Long Island Jewish Medical Center to Dr. Bermanzohn.

Hierarchy, Reductionism, and "Comorbidity" in the Diagnosis of Schizophrenia

Paul C. Bermanzohn, M.D.
Linda Porto, M.S.N., R.N., C.S.
Samuel G. Siris, M.D.
Roz Stronger, M.A.
Michael Y. Hwang, M.D.
Simcha Pollack, Ph.D.

[I]t is very possible that progress in the neurosciences will be severely limited by major shortcomings in descriptive psychiatry.

J. S. Strauss (1994)

*P*sychiatric syndromes appear to co-occur with schizophrenia at substantial rates, but the significance of these findings has remained obscure. The reason for this is, at least in part, that hierarchical conventions have

This work was supported, in part, by a Young Investigator Award from the National Alliance for Research on Schizophrenia and Affective Disorders and a Staff Society grant from the Long Island Jewish Medical Center to Dr. Bermanzohn.

kept these disorders from view. Kept from view, these syndromes have remained unrecognized, undiagnosed, and untreated. Associated psychiatric syndromes (APS) that have been found commonly in patients with schizophrenia and that we consider here include depression (Siris 1991; see also Chapter 2, this volume), obsessive-compulsive disorder (OCD) (Berman et al. 1995a; Fenton and McGlashan 1986; see also Chapter 3, this volume), and panic disorder (Argyle 1990; Boyd 1986; Young et al. 1998; see also Chapter 4, this volume). Yet, despite these replicated findings, surprisingly little work has been done to establish their clinical validity or "practical utility" (Kendell 1989).

Of special concern to clinicians is that, with the exception of depression, few studies have examined the treatability of APS in patients with schizophrenia. Conclusive studies of the treatability of APS have not been done even though it is generally accepted that in the absence of schizophrenia both panic disorder (Barlow et al. 1989) and OCD (Greist et al. 1995a, 1995b) are safely and effectively treatable. Findings from small preliminary studies suggest that panic attacks (Kahn et al. 1988) and OCD (Berman et al. 1995b) in the presence of schizophrenia may be treatable as well.

APS in schizophrenia also may be a source of disability for patients with schizophrenia (Cheadle et al. 1978; Zarate 1997). Thus, we have a situation that would be expected to excite a good deal of medical interest: seemingly common disabling conditions for which treatments may be available. Yet only a small number of preliminary studies have been done to test the treatability of panic symptoms and OCD in patients with schizophrenia.

We suggest here that the conventional systems of diagnosis, with their hierarchical assumptions, have played a role in diverting attention from these syndromes. In DSM-III (American Psychiatric Association 1980), the diagnostic criteria prohibited diagnosis of a number of anxiety and depressive disorders in the presence of schizophrenia. DSM-IV (American Psychiatric Association 1994) has made some progress in recognizing these syndromes, but remnants of the old system persist. These remnants may continue to interfere with the recognition of APS and with their study.

The basic assumption shared by hierarchical systems is that there is a hierarchy of diagnoses and that diagnoses that are higher on the hierarchy subsume diagnoses lower on the hierarchy; this means that the diagnosis of schizophrenia could somehow "explain" or "account for" the presence of lower diagnoses like anxiety disorders found in patients who have been diagnosed with schizophrenia. This assumption is connected to *diagnostic reductionism,* the tendency to reduce all of the symptoms and signs shown by persons with schizophrenia to the schizophrenia alone. Such reductionism undoubtedly contributes to the widespread tendency to treat schizophrenia as if it were a single, unitary disorder.

To illuminate the problems in recognizing APS, we look at the epidemiology of APS in schizophrenia. We then discuss how hierarchical concepts keep APS hidden from clinical and scientific attention. We next address what has been found in those few treatment studies of APS in schizophrenia. We focus especially on panic symptoms and OCD. Since depression has been fairly extensively studied, it may serve as a model for the study of other APS (see Chapter 2, this volume). Finally, we suggest that APS might play a role in the development of a more clinically based system of subclassifying schizophrenia.

Epidemiology

APS have been observed in patients with schizophrenia for many years. Although reported prevalence rates have varied considerably, some estimates have been substantial (Table 1–1). Rates of APS in patients with schizophrenia have been reported several at once (e.g., Bland et al. 1987; Boyd et al. 1984) or one at a time. Soni et al. (1992) found that schizophrenia patients in the community had more depression and anxiety than those in the hospital and attributed this to greater stress on those living in the community.

Differences in the definitions of disorders, in sampling, and in study design account for much of the variability in reported prevalences of APS in schizophrenia. But other factors, especially professional preconceptions based on hierarchical notions of diagnosis, may help explain why APS have only slowly been recognized despite their seemingly substantial prevalence.

Bland et al. (1987) found that 85% of schizophrenia patients (17 of 20) in a randomized community sample had one or more of three APS (i.e., depression, OCD, and panic disorder). The lifetime rates of depression, OCD, and panic disorder were 54.2%, 59.2%, and 29.5%, respectively. Bermanzohn et al. (2000) found that 76% (28 of 37) of an intensively studied sample of chronic schizophrenia patients had symptoms of one or more of these three APS; 48.6% had one or more of the full syndromes. The lifetime rates of depressive disorders, OCD, and panic disorder were 45.9% ($n = 17$), 29.7% ($n = 11$), and 10.8% ($n = 4$), respectively. Although many of these diagnoses were made in violation of the exclusion rules, a number of patients improved when they were openly treated for these conditions with an agent appropriate to the excluded diagnosis.

Depression

The prevalence rates of depression in patients with schizophrenia have varied widely across studies. Siris (1991; see also Chapter 2, this volume), in reviewing the literature on depression in schizophrenia, estimated that the modal prevalence of depression in schizophrenia is about 25%, with rates ranging from 7% to 75%.

Recognition of depression in patients with schizophrenia may be affected in several ways. Depression may be clinically indistinguishable from akinesia or akathisia, two extrapyramidal side effects of neuroleptics (Bermanzohn and Siris 1992; Rifkin et al. 1975; Siris et al. 1987; Van Putten 1975; Van Putten and May 1978). Depression also shares many features (e.g., anhedonia, anergia, and diminished affective expression) with the negative symptoms of schizophrenia (Bermanzohn and Siris 1992; Carpenter et al. 1985a, 1988). Negative symptoms of schizophrenia constitute a class of disturbances considered by many to be inherent in, and fundamental to, the schizophrenic disease process. The psychosocial syndrome of demoralization also may be difficult to distinguish from depression in patients with schizophrenia (de Figueiredo 1993). Whether a study recognized these potential confounds and how it attempted to exclude them may account for much of the variability in reported prevalence rates. These clinical similarities have given rise not only to significant clinical confounds (Siris 1991; Siris et al. 1988) but also to theoretical questions about the very possibility of studying phenomena that are clinically very difficult to distinguish from one another (Lewine and Sommers 1985).

Schizoaffective Disorder

Many cases of depression in patients with schizophrenia are given the label schizoaffective disorder, but the concept of schizoaffective disorder has, in some important respects, been clouded with uncertainty. Levitt and Tsuang (1988) reviewed the literature on schizoaffective disorder and recounted the history of the concept. Kasanin (1933) first used the term *schizoaffective* in describing a group of patients in whom "[t]he psychosis lasts a few weeks to a few months and is followed by a recovery." Vaillant (1964) later studied schizophrenia patients who "recovered"—that is, those who, although they might experience relapses, had a full remission of symptoms and returned to their premorbid level of functioning.

Vaillant (1964) and Stephens et al. (1966) described a series of factors that enabled them to accurately predict remission vs. nonremission in about 80% of the cases. Prominent among these predictors was the presence of depression or "affective symptoms." Thus, the presence of "affective

Table 1-1. Prevalence rates of co-occurring syndromes in schizophrenia

Study	Sample/criteria employed	Findings
	Several APS together	
Cheadle et al. 1978	190 schizophrenia patients living in the community. Pre-DSM categories used.	65.3% ($n = 124$) with "neurotic" symptoms "(almost exclusively) associated with . . . social handicaps, e.g., isolation, unemployment."
Boyd et al. 1984[a]	Epidemiological study of community sample in five U.S. cities. DIS/DSM-III criteria used.	OCD: 12.3 Depression: 28.5 Panic: 37.9
Bland et al. 1987	Random community sample in Edmonton, Alberta, Canada. DIS/DSM-III criteria used.	OCD: 59.2% ($P < 0.01$) Depression: 54.2% ($P < 0.001$) Panic: 29.5% ($P < 0.001$)
Garvey et al. 1991	95 psychiatric inpatients assessed for coexisting anxiety disorders; 18 with schizophrenia based on DSM-III criteria.	Comorbid anxiety in 44%, panic disorder in 17%, GAD in 22% of schizophrenia patients. Results did not support validity of primary/secondary distinction as it pertains to anxiety disorders. Patients with comorbidity may have better prognosis.
Soni et al. 1992	Hospitalized patients with chronic schizophrenia ($n = 201$) compared with matched sample living in the community ($n = 142$); all subjects over age 40 years. Diagnoses based on RDC.[b]	Hospitalized patients were more disorganized and had more negative symptoms of schizophrenia. Community patients had more anxiety and depression.
Strakowski et al. 1993[c]	102 acutely psychotic, hospitalized first-episode patients; 10 patients with disorders in schizophrenia spectrum	OCD: 13.7% Panic: 6.0% Comorbidity in schizophrenia spectrum was associated with longer hospitalization.

Table 1–1. Prevalence rates of co-occurring syndromes in schizophrenia *(continued)*

Study	Sample/criteria employed	Findings
Zarate 1997[d]	60 randomly selected outpatients with schizophrenia or schizoaffective disorder (32 without comorbidity and 28 with comorbidity). DSM-IV criteria used.	OCD: 6.67 Panic disorder: 19.4 56.7% met criteria for lifetime anxiety disorders. Work and overall function were worse in the comorbid group.
Cassano et al. 1998[c]	96 consecutively hospitalized, currently psychotic patients (31 with "schizophrenia spectrum" disorders and 10 with schizophrenia).	OCD: 29% Panic: 19.4% 58.1% of those with schizophrenia spectrum disorder had "comorbidity."
Panic symptoms only		
Boyd 1986	5 large community samples (total $N = 18,572$) as part of ECA survey. DIS/DSM-III criteria used.	28%–63% of subjects with schizophrenia reported panic attacks, depending on the community.
Argyle 1990	20 consecutive patients attending an outpatient clinic for maintenance treatment of chronic schizophrenia. DSM-III-R criteria used.	7 patients (35%) had regularly occurring panic attacks; 4 of these 7 patients (20%) met full criteria for panic disorder. Agoraphobia was present in 3 of the patients with panic attacks and in 1 without panic. Among the 13 patients with significant social avoidance, 4 (20% of the total sample) had typical social phobia, with fears of appearing anxious and being humiliated.
Cutler and Siris 1991	45 patients, mostly outpatients with schizophrenia or schizoaffective disorder who also had operationally defined postpsychotic depression. RDC criteria used.[b]	11 patients (nearly 25%) had panic attacks, as defined by RDC criteria. Number of patients meeting full criteria for panic disorder was not reported.

Table 1-1. Prevalence rates of co-occurring syndromes in schizophrenia (*continued*)

Study	Sample/criteria employed	Findings
Young et al. 1998	54 consecutively admitted VA patients. DSM-IV criteria used.	22 patients (44%) had panic attacks, and 16 (32%) had panic disorder. Patients with paranoid subtype were more likely than patients with schizoaffective or undifferentiated subtype to have had panic attacks or disorder.
OCD only		
Jahrreiss 1926	Chart review of 1,000 hospitalized and clinic patients. Strict criteria for OCD (similar to those in DSM-IV), but not for schizophrenia, used.	11 patients met criteria for OCD; prevalence rate of 11%.
Rosen 1957	Chart review of 848 hospitalized patients. Criteria not specified for either OCD or schizophrenia.	30 patients (3.5%) had OCD "at some time."
Fenton and McGlashan 1986	Follow-up of 163 hospitalized patients. Chart review with follow-up an average of 15 years later. DSM-III-R criteria for schizophrenia used, with behavioral criteria for obsessive-compulsive symptoms.	21 patients (12.9%) met two of eight behavioral criteria for obsessive-compulsive symptoms.
Bland et al. 1987	Random community survey of 2,144 community residents; 20 with schizophrenia. DIS/DSM-III criteria used.	11 patients met DIS/DSM-III criteria for OCD (statistically corrected to 59.2%).

Table 1–1. Prevalence rates of co-occurring syndromes in schizophrenia (*continued*)

Study	Sample/criteria employed	Findings
Berman et al. 1995a	Structured interviews of therapists at CMHC. Therapists of 108 CMHC patients with chronic schizophrenia interviewed. Chart diagnoses used for schizophrenia, and criteria of Fenton and McGlashan (1986) used for obsessive-compulsive symptoms.	27 patients exhibited obsessive-compulsive symptoms during study (point prevalence of 26.5%); 33 patients had obsessive-compulsive symptoms at any time (lifetime prevalence: 30.6%).
D. S. Rae, unpublished data, 1998	Reanalysis of ECA survey data (random community survey of five U.S. communities). DIS/DSM-III criteria used.	OCD: 23.7%
Porto et al. 1997	Lifetime prevalence study, using SCID-IV, of schizophrenia and schizoaffective patients with obsessive-compulsive symptoms and OCD. 50 chronic schizophrenia patients in comprehensive day program interviewed.	"Clinically significant" obsessive-compulsive symptoms: 60% (*n* = 30) Full OCD: 26%
Eisen et al. 1997	Lifetime prevalence study using SCID-III-R. 77 outpatients with schizophrenia or schizoaffective disorder. DSM-III-R criteria used.	6 patients (7.8%) met DSM-III-R criteria for both OCD and schizophrenia.

Table 1–1. Prevalence rates of co-occurring syndromes in schizophrenia *(continued)*

Study	Sample/criteria employed	Findings
Meghani et al. 1998	All new admissions to an outpatient psychiatry service in a large midwestern teaching hospital over 5 years ($N = 1,458$) given structured diagnostic instrument and self-report measures. Criteria unspecified.	31.7% ($n = 61$) of all schizophrenia patients ($N = 192$) met criteria for OCD. Patients with both OCD and schizophrenia had "less efficient psychosocial functioning . . . and lower self-satisfaction." No treatment differences between the two groups were noted except that patients with both OCD and schizophrenia were more likely to say that the medications they received "made no difference."

Note. CMHC = community mental health center; DIS = Diagnostic Interview Schedule; ECA = Epidemiologic Catchment Area; GAD = generalized anxiety disorder; OCD = obsessive-compulsive disorder; RDC = Research Diagnostic Criteria; SCID-III-R = Structured Clinical Interview for DSM-III-R Disorders; SCID-IV = Structured Clinical Interview for DSM-IV Disorders; VA = Veterans Affairs medical center.

[a]Data of Boyd et al. (1984) were presented as odds ratios, not as percentages.

[b]Spitzer et al. 1975.

[c]Depression category not reported because all psychotic disorders, including major depression, were studied.

[d]Data on depression not reported.

symptoms" in schizophrenia patients came to be associated with good outcome of or recovery from schizophrenia. Fowler (1978) referred to schizoaffective disorder as "good-prognosis schizophrenia." On the other hand, Harrow et al. (1998), in a long-term, prospective study, found that schizophrenia patients with posthospital depression showed poorer work functioning and poorer overall adjustment. They also found that depression in patients with schizophrenia was associated with recurrent psychosis.

The category of schizoaffective disorder has been subject to much debate. Whereas some investigators (e.g., Fowler 1978; Levitt and Tsuang 1988) have suggested that it is a heterogeneous mix of disorders, others have viewed it as a subtype of either schizophrenia or affective illness. These divergent views have contributed to a lack of clarity regarding schizoaffective disorder in the diagnostic nosologies. DSM-III included schizoaffective disorder as a diagnosis without any criteria—the only category treated this way—because there was "no consensus on how this category should be defined" (American Psychiatric Association 1980, p. 202). DSM-IV, too, left schizoaffective disorder unclear by defining it as a disorder in which the patient meets criterion A (symptom criterion) for schizophrenia and affective symptoms are present for "a sustantial proportion of the total duration . . . of the illness" (American Psychiatric Association 1994, p. 296). What constitutes "a substantial proportion" is not specified. Thus, where schizoaffective disorder ends and "depression superimposed on schizophrenia" begins is not defined.

Still, depression is the most extensively studied of the APS in schizophrenia (Harrow et al. 1998; Siris et al. 1987, 1994), and much of what has been learned from this work may serve as a model for the study of other APS (for review, see Chapter 2, this volume).

Obsessive-Compulsive Symptoms

Obsessive-compulsive symptoms have been recognized in patients with schizophrenia for many years, but there has been little agreement about how prevalent they are. (A fuller discussion of this topic may be found in Chapter 3 of this volume.) Prevalence estimates of obsessive-compulsive symptoms in schizophrenia have ranged from 1.1% (Jahrreiss 1926) to 59.2% (Bland et al. 1987), and recent studies have tended toward the higher estimates. Different samples were studied in the various investigations and different definitions of OCD and of schizophrenia were used, which probably explains some of the great variability in estimates. This is only a partial explanation, because these symptoms may become intertwined with the psychotic symptoms of schizophrenia, and such phenomenologic overlap may affect estimates of the prevalence of obsessive-compulsive symptoms in schizophrenia (Bermanzohn et al. 1997a).

OCD and schizophrenia overlap phenomenologically because both psychotic delusions and obsessions rest on irrational or excessive ideas. Most OCD patients in whom there is no question of their having schizophrenia retain insight into the absurd or pathological nature of their preoccupations. Yet persons with OCD alone commonly experience some degree of loss of insight into the extreme or senseless nature of their ideas. When this loss of insight is complete or constant, the disorder is referred to as "psychotic OCD" (Insel and Akiskal 1986; Solyom et al. 1985). In persons with schizophrenia, psychotic OCD would be difficult to distinguish clinically from schizophrenic delusions. Moreover, obsessive delusions—hybrid symptoms that are obsessive in form and delusional in content—have been reported to occur in 21.6% of patients with chronic schizophrenia (Bermanzohn et al. 1997b).

Obsessive-compulsive symptoms have been found in schizophrenia patients whose symptoms are refractory to antipsychotic therapy. Some of the treatment resistance these patients exhibit may come from their obsessive symptoms' being viewed as psychotic schizophrenic symptoms that are refractory to antipsychotic medication. Bermanzohn et al. (1997a) reported a case series in which some of these misidentified obsessional symptoms appeared to respond to antiobsessional treatments.

Anxiety, Panic, and Social Phobia

Anxiety is common in patients with schizophrenia. The assessment of anxiety in patients with schizophrenia may be affected in two opposite ways by patients' being administered neuroleptics. Typical neuroleptics commonly cause akathisia—a side effect characterized by a subjective and objective restlessness that can be difficult to distinguish from anxiety (Van Putten 1975)—and so might affect efforts to assess for the presence of panic attacks. Neuroleptics also may have anxiolytic activity, so that some patients receiving neuroleptics may in effect be receiving treatment for their anxiety symptoms (Brauzer et al. 1974; Mendels et al. 1986; Mirabi et al. 1978; Rickels et al. 1972, 1974; Villalobos 1978).

Boyd (1986), describing the results of the Epidemiologic Catchment Area (ECA) study, reported that in the five cities where the ECA was conducted, the frequency of panic attacks in people with schizophrenia ranged from 28% to 63%. Cutler and Siris (1991) found that 24.4% (11 of 45) of their patients with schizophrenia and schizoaffective disorder who presented with postpsychotic depression experienced panic attacks. Argyle

(1990) interviewed 20 consecutive patients with chronic schizophrenia in an outpatient clinic and found that 7 (35%) had panic attacks; 4 of these patients (20%) met the DSM-III-R (American Psychiatric Association 1987) criteria for panic disorder. In his detailed descriptions, Argyle noted that the relationship between panic attacks and psychosis appeared to be complex and variable; in some cases psychosis preceded panic, whereas in other cases the sequence was reversed. Bland et al. (1987), who found panic attacks in 7 of 20 schizophrenia patients (35%, statistically corrected to 29.5%), reported that the panic attacks developed first or simultaneously with the onset of schizophrenia in all 7.

We know of no studies examining the effect of panic symptoms on functional outcome or prognosis in patients with schizophrenia. However, Tien and Eaton (1992), in their examination of the ECA data, found that panic symptoms and social phobia weakly predicted subsequent development of schizophrenia; this association did not reach statistical significance ($P = 0.062$). Heun and Maier (1995) estimated that the risk for schizophrenia in patients with panic disorder is more than 10-fold that in the general population.

Although there have been studies of social performance anxiety in patients with schizophrenia (Penn et al. 1994), few studies have examined the frequency with which social phobia occurs in patients with schizophrenia. Liebowitz et al. (1985), in their review of social phobia, noted that "schizophrenics may at times appear socially phobic, but their social anxieties can logically be attributed to the primary disorder. However, the commonalities of social anxiety in the schizophrenic and nonschizophrenic population remain to be assessed" (p. 730). Social phobia, in which persons may feel unliked or picked on, may be difficult to distinguish from paranoia. Therefore, the assessment of social phobia in patients with schizophrenia is particularly difficult. Since Liebowitz et al.'s review, several investigators have reported social phobia in patients with schizophrenia: 20% of the patients in Argyle's (1990) sample met the criteria for social phobia, and 30% of the patients in Zarate's (1997) sample were diagnosed with social phobia. Bermanzohn (1998) noted that social phobia and paranoia may be confounded in patients with schizophrenia because both entail a fear of others.

Hierarchical Diagnosis and Associated Psychiatric Syndromes

Several studies have found substantial rates of APS in patients with schizophrenia. Some of these studies looked at several APS at once (e.g., Bermanzohn et al. 1995; Bland et al. 1987; Boyd et al. 1984), and others examined individual APS such as panic (e.g., Boyd 1986), OCD (Berman et al. 1995a; Fenton and McGlashan 1986), and depression (Siris 1991; see also Chapter 2, this volume). Although there appears to be agreement that such phenomena are common, their significance remains elusive, in large part because it has been obscured by hierarchical notions of diagnosis. By excluding diagnosis of these disorders, the hierarchical system has prevented their study and so hampered attempts to assess their clinical validity. This lack of clarity concerning their validity promotes the (untested) assumption that APS are of little clinical importance, perhaps merely artifacts of the diagnostic system. In this way, the hierarchical system of diagnosis could become a circular, self-reinforcing system of thought.

Bland et al. (1987) suggested ways in which the clinical significance of APS may be explored (discussed later in this section). But despite the seeming ubiquity of APS in schizophrenia, few studies have examined these questions. Why is this?

Diagnostic reductionism seems to be an important obstacle to recognition and study of psychopathological syndromes that may co-occur with schizophrenia. *Diagnostic reductionism* is a habit of thought that attributes all aberrant or distressing thoughts or behaviors that people with schizophrenia may experience or exhibit to the schizophrenia alone. This line of thinking exists in many forms and is common in clinical discourse. It serves as a brake on inquiry. Although it may take many forms, diagnostic reductionism is an integral part of the hierarchical system of diagnosis.

Hierarchy and "Comorbidity"

Hierarchy

Since at least the 17th century, medicine has had the belief that only one disorder may be present in each patient (Boyd et al. 1984; Foucault 1975; Williams and Hadler 1983). This approach, much like Occam's razor, emphasizes parsimony of explanation and thereby may have contributed to the development of medical science, perhaps by simplifying explanations of observed phenomena. On the other hand, hierarchical notions in psychiatric diagnosis may have forced premature closure on diagnostic questions and thereby obscured the presence of multiple syndromes or minimized their potential significance.

Psychiatric hierarchies are embedded in the way clinicians are taught to think. Such hierarchies are generally similar to one another. Psychiatric diagnoses are arranged in a hierarchy in which "any given diagnosis *excludes* the symptoms of all higher members of the hierarchy and *embraces* the symptoms of all lower members" (Surtees and Kendell 1979, p. 438;

emphasis in original). Such hierarchies commonly start with organic brain disorders at the top, followed by schizophrenia and then bipolar disorder, with "neurotic" disorders (anxiety, OCDs, and depression) at the base of the hierarchy.

Jaspers (1923/1972) first noted hierarchy in Kraepelin's system of psychiatric diagnosis and considered it a useful convention that enabled psychiatrists to assign a single diagnosis to each patient, even when patients had symptoms of various disorders. This hierarchical approach provided a parsimony of diagnosis. Kurt Schneider's (1950) system for diagnosing schizophrenia based on "first rank symptoms" is also a hierarchical system.

On the other hand, hierarchies also may define an important natural sequence in which more common symptoms, such as anxiety and depression, occur first and remit last in the development of a psychiatric disorder. Other symptoms, such as phobic anxiety, anhedonia, and psychomotor retardation, occur less often and rarely without a disturbance of mood, such as anxiety or depression. Finally, psychotic symptoms such as delusions, hallucinations, and disorganized speech are generally the last to develop and the first to remit. The study of prodromal symptoms in schizophrenia (e.g., Herz and Melville 1980; Yung and McGorry 1996), with anxiety and depression typically developing first, might be taken as support for the hierarchical view.

Foulds and Bedford (1975) proposed a slightly different hierarchical model of personal illness. Ignoring organic brain disorders, they identified four classes of psychiatric symptoms (listed from higher to lower): 1) delusions of disintegration, 2) integrated delusions, 3) neurotic symptoms (obsessional, phobic, and hysterical), and 4) dysthymic states (anxiety, depression, and elation). They predicted that psychiatric patients almost always would have symptoms of disorders lower on the hierarchy. Several studies have supported this hypothesis (Bagshaw 1977; Bedford and Presly 1978; Boyd et al. 1984; McPherson et al. 1977; Palmer et al. 1981), whereas others have not (Bagshaw and McPherson 1978; Surtees and Kendell 1979).

DSM-III formalized a hierarchical approach by incorporating various exclusion rules, particularly for schizophrenia. It was assumed that schizophrenia, at the top of the hierarchy of diagnosis, would manifest many of the symptoms of disorders lower on the hierarchy. Hence, several anxiety and depressive disorders could not be diagnosed in the presence of schizophrenia.

This approach caused difficulty for the clinician. Generally, these exclusion rules required that the lower disorder (e.g., anxiety disorder) not be due to a disorder higher on the hierarchy (e.g., schizophrenia) if the lower disorder was to be diagnosed. How to determine that a set of symptoms was "not due to" another disorder was never made clear; such a determination was, at best, difficult to make. In practice, the lower diagnosis was often assumed to be "due to" the higher diagnosis. Anxiety and depressive disorders often were not diagnosed in the presence of schizophrenia but in effect were absorbed into it.

This system also created similar dilemmas for the psychiatric epidemiologist. In epidemiologic studies, it was "difficult to determine whether low (or high) rates of a particular disorder were due to correspondingly high (or low) rates of an excluding disorder, rather than to variation in the rate for the original disorder" (Bland et al. 1987, p. 384). As a result, studies have reported coexisting APS in persons with schizophrenia on the basis of "non-hierarchical" diagnoses (Bland et al. 1987; Boyd et al. 1984).

The studies based on nonhierarchical diagnoses generally have found substantial rates of APS in patients with schizophrenia, yet they also have been unclear as to the significance of APS. Bland et al. (1987) suggested that "[t]he practical significance of co-morbidity must be demonstrated in studies examining outcome differentials and co-morbidity patterns (e.g., schizophrenics with and without obsessional symptoms), family studies demonstrating differential morbidity risk according to patterns of co-morbidity . . . and showing that differential treatment responses are associated with patterns of co-morbidity" (p. 389). Boyd et al. (1984), using ECA survey data, found highly significant relationships between a diagnosis of schizophrenia and "excluded disorders"[1]—disorders that, according to DSM-III, were excluded by a diagnosis of schizophrenia. Although Boyd et al. recognized this was "an operating assumption of DSM-III that has not received the kind of empirical research it deserves" (p. 989), the only suggestion they made about how to investigate the clinical significance of these widespread phenomena was to do follow-up studies. They proposed that if the presence of these excluded disorders made no difference in the long-term outcome of the excluding disorder, this would support the hierarchical system. This line of reasoning is similar to one of the three parts of

---

[1]Boyd et al. (1984) reported their data in terms of odds ratios and did not give the frequencies of co-occurring syndromes. This makes comparison with our data (Bermanzohn et al. 2000) and those of Bland et al. (1987) difficult. They also studied depression as an "excluding disorder." There are many interesting parallels between depression and schizophrenia and their problems with "excluded" disorders, such as how one should interpret the high rates of panic disorder in depression.

a research plan proposed by Bland et al. (1987) but is not an adequate plan by itself. Boyd et al. (1984) considered their findings largely as a confirmation of the hierarchical system.

DSM-IV and Hierarchical Exclusions

DSM-IV now permits multiple diagnoses on Axis I—an approach that has opened the way for many studies of psychiatric "comorbidity." But many remnants of the hierarchical system remain in DSM-IV (Bermanzohn et al. 2000), which now generally requires that a lower disorder be "not better accounted for" by a higher disorder. This statement of exclusion—"not better accounted for"—is only marginally different from that represented by the wording "not due to" in DSM-III-R. Like its predecessor, DSM-IV gives no guidance as to how to determine that some symptoms are "not better accounted for" or "not due to" another disorder. In at least some cases, the natural tendency is to fall back on old patterns and to fail to recognize or even look for APS in patients with schizophrenia.

On Names and Terms

Psychopathological syndromes co-occurring with schizophrenia have been described in the literature with a variety of names, including "comorbid conditions" (with the co-occurrence called "comorbidity") (Bland et al. 1987; Hwang and Opler 1994; Strakowski et al. 1993), "secondary syndromes" (Siris 1993; Winokur 1988), "hierarchy-free" or "non-hierarchical" syndromes (Boyd et al. 1984), and "Associated Psychiatric Syndromes" (Bermanzohn et al. 1995). They are also referred to with terms formed by appending the prefix "schizo-" to the name of the syndrome, such as "schizodepressive," "schizo-obsessive," "schizomanic," and "schizopanic." Some of these approaches to naming these disorders appear to reflect unwarranted assumptions about the nature of the syndromes being described and may cause confusion.

The most commonly used term, *comorbidity*, generally refers to the co-occurrence of two or more separate disorders with distinct or overlapping etiologies. But in the case of schizophrenia and its co-occurring syndromes, no etiology has been proven. Indeed, whether these are separate disorders or dimensions of the schizophrenia itself (Hwang and Opler 1994) is unresolved. Use of this term in schizophrenia seems to go beyond what is known. Use of the prefix "schizo-" to designate co-occurring syndromes when they are present simultaneously with schizophrenia seems to invite the lack of clarity that has been associated with the term schizoaffective.

The term *secondary syndromes* may have two meanings: either the designated syndrome appears after the schizophrenia ("secondary" used to mean "later") or the syndrome causes less morbidity than the schizophrenia ("secondary" used to mean "subordinate" to the schizophrenia or "less" damaging to the patient). Neither usage appears warranted in light of what is known about these syndromes. First, in reports that have looked at obsessive-compulsive and panic symptoms in schizophrenia, these co-occurring symptoms generally have preceded the onset of the schizophrenia (Argyle 1990; Bermanzohn et al. 2000; Bland et al. 1987; Fenton and McGlashan 1986). Second, in the chronic patients studied by Cheadle et al. (1978), much of the disability was concentrated among those with "neurotic disorders"—disorders that are similar to the syndromes under discussion here. Our clinical experience also suggests that for some schizophrenia patients whose psychosis is well controlled by antipsychotic medications, the co-occurring psychopathology may be the principal, not a lesser or "secondary," source of disability. Zarate (1997) reported that schizophrenia patients with "comorbid" anxiety disorders exhibited worse work and overall functioning.

The terms *nonhierarchical* and *hierarchy-free* are accurate and useful when applied to the domain of nosology, but they do not provide any information about the clinical expression of co-occurring syndromes. For these reasons, we refer to these co-occurring syndromes as associated psychiatric syndromes, or APS. This term, while unwieldy and awkward, seems best at this time because it does not suggest any particular relationship between the schizophrenia and the co-occurring syndrome other than to say they are associated in some way. And, as Bland et al. (1987) pointed out, it appears that APS may occur in people with schizophrenia more frequently than they occur in the general population.

Clinical "Common Sense" and Hierarchical Notions

Clinicians also often dismiss evidence of APS. These dismissals may appear to be simple common sense, but these "commonsense" ideas rest on hierarchical notions. These sentiments appear to be widespread, given that their expression is so commonly encountered in clinical discourse.

Dismissals of evidence of APS occur in a variety of ways. On noting depression in a patient with schizophrenia, a clinician is likely to remark, "She has a lot to be depressed about, since she's schizophrenic." Similarly, on observing severe anxiety in a patient with schizophrenia, the clinician may comment, "Who wouldn't be anxious if they believed they are being followed?" Finally, if a schizophrenia patient can't stop talking about a delusion, the clinician is likely to describe this as "such a severe psychotic symptom that he can't stop thinking and talking about it." In someone without schizophrenia, the inability to stop thinking some thought or endlessly repeating it would suggest the possibility of an obsessive disorder. In each of these three cases, the problem is attributed to the schizophrenia alone, as if no other disturbance (or dimension of disturbance) were present. This is perhaps the clearest expression of diagnostic reductionism, reflecting the hierarchical assumptions we are taught about schizophrenia. Such tacit assumptions stand in the way of recognizing APS.

Validity of "Lower" Disorders: Prognosis, Treatability, and Heritability

Although disorders lower in the hierarchy may be dismissed or even ignored, it has been unclear what the significance of these disorders might be. To address this issue, Bland et al. (1987) proposed a research agenda that included the relation of these disorders to prognosis, treatability, and heritability. Data from studies of depression, obsessive-compulsive symptoms, and panic in persons with schizophrenia suggest that disorders lower on the hierarchy may be relevant both to clinical treatment and to the prediction of course of illness and outcome in patients with schizophrenia. Whereas the relation of depression to schizophrenia has been fairly well studied, few studies have addressed the relation of panic and obsessive-compulsive symptoms to schizophrenia.

Siris et al. (1987, 1994) showed that treating depression in schizophrenia patients led to improvement in the depressive symptoms and protection from psychotic relapse. These findings suggest that treating disorders lower on the hierarchy (e.g., depression) may have clinical significance, even in the presence of a disorder higher on the hierarchy (i.e., schizophrenia). Siris et al.'s (1987) findings also suggest that antidepressant medication (specifically imipramine) may be safely and efficaciously used in clinically stable patients with chronic schizophrenia who are not flagrantly psychotic. This has possible relevance for the treatment of both panic symptoms and OCD, in which the chief pharmacological agents are antidepressant medicines.

Harrow et al. (1998) presented data from their prospective follow-up studies of depression in patients with schizophrenia 4.5 and 7 years after an index admission. These data suggested that the presence of depression is associated with poor outcome and disability in patients with schizophrenia. Parallel questions may be asked: What role do OCD and panic symptoms play in the course and outcome of schizophrenia, and could treatment influence these outcomes?

Obsessive-compulsive symptoms appear to play a role in the course and outcome of schizophrenia. In their longitudinal study of Chestnut Lodge patients with schizophrenia, Fenton and McGlashan (1986) found that those with obsessive-compulsive symptoms ($n = 21$) had a worse prognosis than those without such symptoms ($n = 142$). Berman et al. (1995b) confirmed these findings by interviewing the therapists of 108 chronic schizophrenia patients about the patients' symptoms and ability to function. Samuels et al. (1993) likewise found that schizophrenia patients with obsessive-compulsive symptoms had more florid symptoms, an earlier age at onset of psychosis, an earlier age at first hospitalization, and a greater number of hospitalizations than schizophrenia patients without obsessive-compulsive symptoms. Relatives of schizophrenia patients with obsessive-compulsive symptoms have been found to have higher rates of major depression and suicide than relatives of schizophrenia patients without obsessive-compulsive symptoms (A. E. Pulver, Ph.D., personal communication, 1996). This finding suggests that there may be a familial component to obsessive-compulsive symptoms in schizophrenia and that it is important to distinguish clinical subgroups for etiological and genetic studies of schizophrenia (Samuels et al. 1993). Recently, Green et al. (1998) presented data comparing obsessive-compulsive symptoms in the relatives of probands who had both schizophrenia and OCD with those in the relatives of patients with schizophrenia alone. Their preliminary findings suggest that obsessive-compulsive symptoms and schizophrenia are not separate or "comorbid" disorders.

Given the potential importance of obsessive-compulsive symptoms in schizophrenia, it is disappointing that only five reports of treating schizophrenia patients with obsessive-compulsive symptoms with adjunctive anti-obsessional agents have appeared in the literature (for review, see Bermanzohn, in press; Sasson et al. 1997; Siris et al. 1997). All these reports involved the use of clomipramine, and in only one of the reports (i.e., Berman et al. 1995a) was the trial controlled. There has been only one case report of cognitive-behavioral therapy for obsessive-compulsive symptoms in a patient with hallucinations and delusions (Lelliott and Marks 1987).

There have been no studies of the effect of panic symptoms, despite their reportedly wide prevalence, on outcome in patients with schizophrenia. There have been only a small number of anecdotal reports of the pharmacological treatment of panic symptoms in patients with schizophrenia and only one prospective study—that of Kahn et al. (1988), which was open and uncontrolled (see Chapter 4, this volume, for a review). We are aware of only one report in which cognitive-behavioral therapy was used to treat panic symptoms in a group of patients with schizophrenia ($N = 8$)

(Arlow et al. 1997), even though cognitive-behavioral therapy is considered by some to be the preferred treatment for panic disorder in the absence of schizophrenia (Arlow et al. 1997). These reports, although involving a small number of patients, all yielded positive findings and suggest that treatments for panic symptoms in patients with schizophrenia may be effective and safe. But larger, more definitive treatment studies still need to be done to test this hypothesis.

The lack of studies of phenomena that appear to be widespread among patients with schizophrenia seems to be a consequence of the hierarchical approach to diagnosis. Excluding diagnoses lower on the hierarchy may result in not paying attention to potentially important clinical phenomena. The parsimony of diagnosis provided by the hierarchical system may come at a price to the patient.

Summary of Factors Interfering With Clinical Assessment of APS

Besides being hidden by the hierarchical system of diagnosis, as we have seen, APS are difficult to recognize for several other reasons. First, patients often conceal these syndromes. More than one schizophrenia patient, in discussing the frightening and humiliating symptoms of panic or obsessions, has said, "People might think I'm crazy if I talk about this." Medicine's hierarchical preconceptions may combine with the shame of patients to keep APS concealed, making it difficult to elicit these symptoms in patients with schizophrenia. Second, psychotic symptoms may also interfere with the assessment of APS because they are more dramatic phenomena and thus are judged to be a more urgent clinical priority (Knights and Hirsch 1981). Patients may also psychotically interpret physiological symptoms—that is, they may have idiosyncratic or bizarre interpretations of their bodily experiences and may also communicate these experiences in a distorted manner—thereby making them harder to recognize (Cutler and Siris 1991). Cognitive impairments may limit schizophrenia patients' capacity to recognize and communicate about their experiences. Psychotic symptoms may be present during an active psychotic episode or may be chronically present in the person with schizophrenia. Additionally, negative symptoms may also make it difficult to assess the patient for APS, especially depression (Bermanzohn and Siris 1992; Carpenter et al. 1985a; Rifkin et al. 1975; Siris 1987; Van Putten and May 1978) and possibly social phobia (Argyle 1990; Finkel 1987), because of potentially overlapping features.

Finally, neuroleptic effects may obscure APS. Akathisia may mimic anxiety (Van Putten 1975), interfering with the recognition of panic symptoms. Antipsychotics also have anxiolytic properties, even in persons who are not psychotic (Brauzer et al. 1974; Cutler and Siris 1991; Mendels et al. 1986; Mirabi et al. 1978; Villalobos 1978), so schizophrenia patients, most of whom are taking neuroleptics, actually may be receiving treatment for their anxiety. Akinesia may be indistinguishable from depression, and this can lead to diagnostic difficulties (Siris 1987). Finally, some of the newer antipsychotic agents have been implicated in the provocation of obsessive-compulsive symptoms (Ames et al. 1995; Baker et al. 1992, 1997; Patel and Tandon 1993; Patil 1992; but see also Ghaemi et al. 1995). All these effects create potential clinical confounds that may add to the clinical difficulty in assessing APS.

Potential Implications for Nosology

APS, rather than being ignored, might provide a basis for a new clinically based subtyping system for schizophrenia—one that might be an improvement over the traditional system now in use (Bermanzohn et al. 1998).

Criticisms of Classical Subtypes

Classical subtypes were subjected to a great deal of criticism in the 1970s (McGlashan and Fenton 1991) for being temporally unstable, phenomenologically nonspecific, and of dubious validity (Carpenter and Stephens 1979; Guggenheim and Babigian 1974; Hay and Forrest 1972; Katz et al. 1964; Munoz et al. 1972; Van der Velde 1976). A more recent proposal, based largely on factor-analytic studies, has been to subtype schizophrenia symptoms into negative, positive, and disorganized types (Andreasen et al. 1995).

Pfohl and Winokur (1983) found a persistent tendency toward nonspecificity of subtypes over time. Several studies since then have reported that classical subtypes have only modest diagnostic stability over time, tending to change in the direction of greater disorganization (hebephrenia) or nonspecificity (undifferentiated) in the classical subtypes and a drift toward deficit syndromes in the deficit/nondeficit subtypes (Kendler et al. 1995; Leboyer et al. 1990; McGlashan and Fenton 1993). On the other hand, Parnas et al. (1988) found a high degree of stability in the paranoid/nonparanoid distinction over 6 years among female patients with schizophrenia.

Classical subtypes not only are unstable but, more important for the clinician, provide no treatment guidance. The mainstay of treatment for schizophrenia is antipsychotic medications. Beyond this, there are no specific treatments for particular classical subtypes.

Possible Role of APS in Subtyping

APS have not yet been studied adequately to assess whether they could be a basis for a system of subtyping schizophrenia. However, several observations suggest such a new subtyping system may be possible:

1. *APS are long-lived.* Several investigators have independently noted that the onset of obsessive-compulsive symptoms, when present, usually precedes the onset of schizophrenia (Bland et al. 1987; Fenton and McGlashan 1986; Rosen 1957; Stengel 1945). Panic symptoms, when present comorbidly, were also found to precede the onset of schizophrenia (Bermanzohn et al. 1996; Bland et al. 1987).

2. *APS may affect prognosis.* A number of investigators have reported that obsessive-compulsive symptoms may significantly affect the course of illness (Berman et al. 1995a; Fenton and McGlashan 1986; Rosen 1957; Samuels et al. 1993; Stengel 1945), but the results are not consistent regarding how they affect prognosis. Earlier investigators (Stengel 1945; Rosen 1957) reported that obsessive-compulsive symptoms were associated with a less virulent course of illness and improved outcome. More recent, more systematic studies (Fenton and McGlashan 1986; Samuels et al. 1993; Berman et al. 1995a) found an association between obsessive-compulsive symptoms and a worse functional outcome. Persistent depression also has been found to be associated with a worse functional outcome (Sands and Harrow 1994). These findings have already prompted some authors (e.g., Berman 1998; Bermanzohn et al. 1998; Hwang and Opler 1994; Samuels et al. 1993; Zohar 1997) to propose obsessive-compulsive symptoms as a subtype of schizophrenia. We are not proposing a specific subtype here, but we are suggesting that APS might offer an approach to subtyping schizophrenia.

3. *APS may have implications for treatment.* The details of such treatments and their efficacy remain to be worked out, but these interventions may be based on treatments used in the syndrome when schizophrenia is not part of the clinical picture.

4. *APS appears to have affected a large percentage of schizophrenia patients who were studied for all three syndromes:* 85% in Bland et al.'s (1987) study and 76% in the study by Bermanzohn et al. (2000). These findings suggest that these syndromes may be useful in classifying a large percentage of patients.

These four points suggest that APS potentially could be a useful basis for subtyping schizophrenia and that such a system might offer guidance in treatment planning.

Summary

Although largely ignored, APS appear to be widespread and may explain a portion of the heterogeneity of schizophrenia. We have tried to describe some of the obstacles, both clinical and theoretical, that have made these syndromes difficult to see. It is suggested that APS may play a role in defining a clinical system for subtyping schizophrenia.

References

American Psychiatric Association: Diagnostic and Statistical Manual of Mental Disorders, 3rd Edition. Washington, DC, American Psychiatric Association, 1980

American Psychiatric Association: Diagnostic and Statistical Manual of Mental Disorders, 3rd Edition, Revised. Washington, DC, American Psychiatric Association, 1987

American Psychiatric Association: Diagnostic and Statistical Manual of Mental Disorders, 4th Edition. Washington, DC, American Psychiatric Association, 1994

Ames D, Wirsching WC, Marder SR, et al: Emergent obsessive compulsive and depressive symptoms with risperidone: a controlled prospective study. Poster presentation at the 34th annual meeting of the American College of Neuropsychopharmacology, San Juan, Puerto Rico, December 11–15, 1995

Andreasen NC, Arndt S, Alliger R, et al: Symptoms of schizophrenia: methods, meanings, and mechanisms. Arch Gen Psychiatry 52:341–351, 1995

Argyle N: Panic Attacks in chronic schizophrenia. Br J Psychiatry 157:430–433, 1990

Arlow PB, Moran ME, Bermanzohn PC, et al: Cognitive-behavioral therapy for panic in schizophrenia. J Psychother Pract Res 6:145–150, 1997

Bagshaw VE: A replication study of Foulds' and Bedford's hierarchical model of depression. Br J Psychiatry 131:53–55, 1977

Bagshaw VE, McPherson FM: The applicability of the Foulds and Bedford hierarchy model to mania and hypomania. Br J Psychiatry 132:293–295, 1978

Baker RW, Chengappa KNR, Baird JW, et al: Emergence of obsessive-compulsive symptoms during treatment with clozapine. J Clin Psychiatry 53:439–441, 1992

Baker RW, Bermanzohn PC, Wirsching DA, et al: Obsessions, compulsions clozapine and risperidone. CNS Spectrums 2(3):26–36, 1997

Barlow DH, Craske MG, Cerny JA, et al: Behavioral treatment of panic disorder. Behavior Therapy 20:261–282, 1989

Bedford DA, Presly AS: Symptom patterns among chronic schizophrenic inpatients. Br J Psychiatry 133:176–178, 1978

Berman I: Is there an OC subtype of schizophrenia? Paper presented at the 151st annual meeting of the American Psychiatric Association, Toronto, Ontario, Canada, May 30–June 4, 1998

Berman I, Kalinowski A, Berman SM, et al: Obsessive and compulsive symptoms in chronic schizophrenia. Compr Psychiatry 36:6–10, 1995a

Berman I, Sapers BL, Chang HHJ, et al: Treatment of obsessive-compulsive symptoms in schizophrenic patients with clomipramine. J Clin Psychopharmacology 15:206–210, 1995b

Bermanzohn PC: Is panic a subtype of schizophrenia? Poster presentation at the 151st annual meeting of the American Psychiatric Association, Toronto, Ontario, Canada, May 30–June 4, 1998

Bermanzohn PC: Recognition and treatment of OC symptoms in schizophrenia: a mini-review. Focus on OCD (in press)

Bermanzohn PC, Siris SG: Akinesia: a syndrome common to parkinsonism, retarded depression, and negative symptoms. Compr Psychiatry 33:221–232, 1992

Bermanzohn PC, Porto L, Siris SG: Associated psychiatric syndromes (APS) in chronic schizophrenia. Poster presentation at the 34th annual meeting of the American College of Neuropsychopharmacology, San Juan, Puerto Rico, December 11–15, 1995

Bermanzohn PC, Porto L, Siris SG: Hierarchical diagnosis in schizophrenia, in Proceedings of the 35th Annual Meeting of the American College of Neuropsychopharmacology, San Juan, Puerto Rico, December 9–13, 1996

Bermanzohn PC, Porto L, Arlow PB, et al: Are some neuroleptic-refractory symptoms of schizophrenia really obsessions? CNS Spectrums 2(3):51–57, 1997a

Bermanzohn PC, Porto L, Arlow PB, et al: Obsessions and delusions: separate and distinct, or overlapping? CNS Spectrums 2(3):58–61, 1997b

Bermanzohn PC, Porto L, Siris SG: Associated syndromes in schizophrenia and clinical subtyping. Poster presentation at the 151st annual meeting of the American Psychiatric Association, Toronto, Ontario, Canada, May 30–June 4, 1998

Bermanzohn PC, Porto L, Siris SG, et al: Hierarchical diagnosis in chronic schizophrenia: a clinical study of co-occurring syndromes. Schizophr Bull 26:519–527, 2000

Bland RC, Newman SC, Orn H: Schizophrenia: lifetime comorbidity in a community sample. Acta Psychiatrica Scand 75:383–391, 1987

Boyd JH: Use of mental health services for the treatment of panic disorder. Am J Psychiatry 143:1569–1574, 1986

Boyd JH, Burke JD Jr, Gruenberg E, et al: Exclusion criteria of DSM-III: a study of co-occurrence of hierarchy-free syndromes. Arch Gen Psychiatry 41:983–989, 1984

Brauzer B, Goldstein BJ, Steinbook RM, et al: The treatment of mixed anxiety and depression with loxapine: a controlled comparative study. J Clin Pharmacol 14:455–463, 1974

Carpenter WT Jr, Stephens JH: An attempted integration of information relevant to schizophrenic subtypes. Schizophr Bull 5:490–506, 1979

Carpenter WT Jr, Heinrichs DW, Alphs LD: Treatment of negative symptoms. Schizophr Bull 11:440–452, 1985

Carpenter WT Jr, Heinrichs DW, Wagman AMI: Deficit and nondeficit forms of schizophrenia: the concept. Am J Psychiatry 145:578–583, 1988

Cassano GB, Pini S, Saetonni M, et al: Occurrence and clinical correlates of psychiatric comorbidity in patients with psychotic disorders. J Clin Psychiatry 59:60–68, 1998

Cheadle AJ, Freeman HL, Korer J: Chronic schizophrenic patients in the community. Br J Psychiatry 132:221–227, 1978

Cutler J, Siris SG: "Panic-like" symptomatology in schizophrenic and schizoaffective patients with postpsychotic depression: observations and implications. Compr Psychiatry 32:465–473, 1991

de Figueiredo JM: Depression and demoralization: phenomenologic differences and research perspectives. Compr Psychiatry 34:308–311, 1993

Eisen JL, Beer DA, Pato MT, et al: Obsessive-compulsive disorder in patients with schizophrenia or schizoaffective disorder. Am J Psychiatry 154:271–273, 1997

Fenton WS, McGlashan TH: The prognostic significance of obsessive-compulsive symptoms in schizophrenia. Am J Psychiatry 143:437–441, 1986

Finkel JA: Diazepam in a patient with chronic schizophrenia complicated by agoraphobia. J Clin Psychiatry 48:33–34, 1987

Foucault M: The Birth of the Clinic: An Archeology of Medical Perception. St Paul, MN, Vintage Books, 1975

Foulds GA, Bedford A: Hierarchy of classes of personal illness. Psychol Med 5:181–192, 1975

Fowler RC: Remitting schizophrenia as a variant of affective disorder. Schizophr Bull 4:68–77, 1978

Garvey M, Noyes R Jr, Anderson B, et al: Examination of comorbid anxiety in psychiatric inpatients. Compr Psychiatry 32:277–282, 1991

Ghaemi SN, Zarate CA, Popli AP, et al: Is there a relationship between clozapine and obsessive compulsive disorder? A retrospective chart review. Compr Psychiatry 36:267–270, 1995

Green AI, Faraone SV, Lee H, et al: Obsessive-compulsive symptoms in the relatives of schizophrenia patients. Paper presented at the 151st annual meeting of the American Psychiatric Association, Toronto, Ontario, Canada, May 30–June 4, 1998

Greist JH, Jefferson JW, Kobak KA, et al: Efficacy and tolerability of serotonin transport inhibitors in obsessive-compulsive disorder: a meta-analysis. Arch Gen Psychiatry 52:53–60, 1995a

Greist JH, Jefferson JW, Kobak KA, et al: A 1 year double-blind placebo-controlled fixed dose study of sertraline in the treatment of obsessive-compulsive disorder. Int Clin Psychopharmacology 10:57–65, 1995b

Guggenheim FG, Babigian HM: Diagnostic consistency in catatonic schizophrenia. Schizophr Bull 11:103–198, 1974

Harrow M, Sands JR, Goldberg JF, et al: How vulnerable are schizophrenic patients to depression? Paper presented at the 151st annual meeting of the American Psychiatric Association, Toronto, Ontario, Canada, May 30–June 4, 1998

Hay AJ, Forrest AD: The diagnosis of schizophrenia and paranoid psychosis: an attempt at clarification. Br J Med Psychol 45:233–241, 1972

Herz MI, Melville C: Relapse in schizophrenia. Am J Psychiatry 137:801–805, 1980

Heun R, Maier W: Relationship of schizophrenia and panic disorder: evidence from a controlled family study. Am J Med Genet 60:127–132, 1995

Hwang MY, Opler LA: Schizophrenia with obsessive-compulsive features: assessment and treatment. Psychiatric Annals 24:468–472, 1994

Insel TR, Akiskal HS: OCD with psychotic features: a phenomenologic analysis. Am J Psychiatry 143:1527–1533, 1986

Jahrreiss W: Obsessions during schizophrenia (in German). Archiv für Psychiatrie und Nervenkrankheiten 77:740–788, 1926

Jaspers K: Compulsion phenomena, in General Psychopathology (1923). Translated by Hoenig J, Hamilton MW. Chicago, IL, University of Chicago Press, 1972, pp 133–137

Kahn JP, Puertollano MA, Schane MD, et al: Adjunctive alprazolam for schizophrenia with panic anxiety: clinical observation and pathogenetic implications. Am J Psychiatry 145:742–744, 1988

Kasanin J: The acute schizoaffective psychoses. Am J Psychiatry 90:97–126, 1933

Katz MM, Cole JO, Lowert HA: Non-specificity of diagnosis of paranoid schizophrenia. Arch Gen Psychiatry 11:197–202, 1964

Kendell RE: Clinical validity. Psychol Med 19:45–55, 1989

Kendler KS, McGuire M, Gruenberg AM, et al: Examining the validity of DSM-III-R schizoaffective disorder and its putative subtypes in the Roscommon family study. Am J Psychiatry 152:755–764, 1995

Knights A, Hirsch SA: "Revealed" depression and drug treatment for schizophrenia. Arch Gen Psychiatry 36:806–811, 1981

Leboyer M, Jay M, D'Amato T, et al: Subtyping familial schizophrenia: reliability, concordance, and stability. Psychiatry Res 34:77–88, 1990

Lelliott P, Marks I: Management of obsessive compulsive rituals associated with delusions, hallucinations and depression: a case report. Behavioral Psychotherapy 15:77–87, 1987

Levitt JJ, Tsuang MT: The heterogeneity of schizoaffective disorder: implications for treatment. Am J Psychiatry 145:926-936, 1988

Lewine RJ, Sommers AA: Clinical definition of negative symptoms as a reflection of theory and methodology, in Controversies in Schizophrenia: Changes and Constancies. Edited by Alpert M. New York, Guilford, 1985, pp 267–279

Liebowitz MA, Gorman JM, Fyer AJ, et al: Social phobia: review of a neglected anxiety disorder. Arch Gen Psychiatry 42:729–735, 1985

McGlashan TH, Fenton WF: Classical subtypes for schizophrenia: literature review for DSM-IV. Schizophr Bull 17:609–623, 1991

McPherson FM, Antram MC, Bagshaw VE, et al: A test of the hierarchical model of personal illness. Br J Psychiatry 131:56–68, 1977

Meghani SR, Penick EC, Nickel EJ, et al: Schizophrenia patients with and without OCD. Poster presentation at the 151st annual meeting of the American Psychiatric Association, Toronto, Ontario, Canada, May 30–June 4, 1998

Mendels J, Krajewski TF, Huffer V, et al: Effective short-term treatment of generalized anxiety disorder with trifluoperazine. J Clin Psychiatry 47:170–174, 1986

Mirabi M, Mathew RJ, Claghorn JL: When is a neuroleptic appropriate in psychoneurosis? Current Therapeutics Research 23:101–104, 1978

Munoz RA, Kulak G, Marten S, et al: Simple and hebephrenic schizophrenia: a follow-up study, in Life History Research in Psychopathology, Vol 2. Edited by Roff M, Robbins LN, Pollack M. Minneapolis, University of Minnesota Press, 1972, pp 228–235

Palmer RL, Ekisa EG, Winbow AJ: Patterns of self-reported symptoms in chronic psychiatric patients. Br J Psychiatry 139:209–212, 1981

Parnas J, Jorgensen A, Teasdale TW, et al: Temporal course of symptoms and social functioning in relapsing schizophrenics. Compr Psychiatry 29:361–371, 1988

Patel B, Tandon R: Development of obsessive compulsive symptoms during clozapine treatment (letter). Am J Psychiatry 150:836, 1993

Patil VJ: Development of transient obsessive-compulsive symptoms during treatment with clozapine (letter). Am J Psychiatry 149:272, 1992

Penn DL, Hope DA, Spaulding W, et al: Social anxiety in schizophrenia. Schizophr Res 11:277–284, 1994

Pfohl B, Winokur G: The micropsychopathology of hebephrenic catatonic schizophrenia. J Nerv Ment Dis 171:296–300, 1983

Porto L, Bermanzohn PC, Pollack S, et al: A profile of obsessive-compulsive symptoms in chronic schizophrenia. CNS Spectrums 2(3):26–33, 1997

Rickels K, Hutchison J, Morris RJ, et al: Molindone and chlordiazepoxide in anxious neurotic outpatients. Current Therapeutics Research 14:1–9, 1972

Rickels K, Weise CC, Clark EL, et al: Thiothixene and thioridazine in anxiety. Br J Psychiatry 125:79–87, 1974

Rifkin A, Quitkin F, Klein DF: Akinesia: a poorly recognized drug-induced extrapyramidal disorder. Arch Gen Psychiatry 32:672–675, 1975

Rosen I: The clinical significance of obsessions in schizophrenia. Journal of Mental Science 103:773–788, 1957

Samuels J, Nestadt G, Wolyniec P, et al: Obsessive-compulsive symptoms in schizophrenia (abstract). Schizophr Res (9):139, 1993

Sands JR, Harrow M: Psychotic unipolar depression at follow-up: factors related to psychosis in the affective disorders. Am J Psychiatry 151:995–1000, 1994

Sasson Y, Bermanzohn PC, Zohar J: Treatment of obsessive-compulsive syndromes in schizophrenia. CNS Spectrums 2(4):34–45, 1997

Schneider K: Clinical Psychopathology. New York, Grune & Stratton, 1950

Siris SG: Adjunctive medication in the maintenance treatment of schizophrenia and its conceptual implications. Br J Psychiatry 163(suppl 22):66–78, 1993

Siris SG: Akinesia and postpsychotic depression: a difficult differential diagnosis. J Clin Psychiatry 48:240–243, 1987

Siris SG: Diagnosis of secondary depression in schizophrenia: implications for DSM-IV. Schizophr Bull 17:75–98, 1991

Siris SG: Adjunctive medication in the maintenance treatment of schizophrenia and its conceptual implications. Br J Psychiatry 163 (suppl 22):66–78, 1993

Siris SG, Morgan V, Fagerstrom R, et al: Adjunctive imipramine in the treatment of postpsychotic depression: a controlled trial. Arch Gen Psychiatry 44:533–539, 1987

Siris SG, Adan F, Cohen M, et al: Post-psychotic depression and negative symptoms: an investigation of syndromal overlap. Am J Psychiatry 145:1532–1537, 1988

Siris SG, Bermanzohn PC, Mason SE, et al: Maintenance imipramine for secondary depression in schizophrenia: a controlled trial. Arch Gen Psychiatry 51:109–115, 1994

Siris SG, Bermanzohn PC, Kessler RJ, et al: Drug treatment of schizophrenia with comorbidity, in Treatment Strategies for Patients With Psychiatric Comorbidity. Edited by Wetzler S, Sanderson WC. New York, Wiley, 1997, pp 219–252

Solyom L, DiNicola VF, Sookman D, et al: Is there an obsessive psychosis? Aetiological and prognostic factors of an atypical form of obsessive compulsive neurosis. Can J Psychiatry 30:372–379, 1985

Soni SD, Mallik A, Reed P, et al: Differences between chronic schizophrenic patients in the hospital and in the community. Hospital and Community Psychiatry 43:1233–1238, 1992

Spitzer RL, Endicott J, Robins E: Research diagnostic criteria. Psychopharmacol Bull 11:22–25, 1975

Stengel E: A study on some clinical aspects of the relationship between obsessional neurosis and psychotic reaction types. Journal of Mental Science 91:166–187, 1945

Stephens JA, Astrup C, Mangrum JC: Prognostic factors in recovered and deteriorated schizophrenics. Am J Psychiatry 122:1116–1121, 1966

Strakowski SM, Tohen M, Stoll AL, et al: Comorbidity in psychosis at first hospitalization. Am J Psychiatry 150:752–757, 1993

Strauss JS: Is biological psychiatry building on an adequate base? Clinical realities and underlying processes in schizophrenic disorders, in Schizophrenia: From Mind to Molecule. Edited by Andreasen NC. Washington, DC, American Psychiatric Press, 1994, pp 31–44

Surtees PG, Kendell RE: The hierarchy model of psychiatric symptomatology: an investigation based on Present State Examination ratings. Br J Psychiatry 135:438–443, 1979

Tien AY, Eaton WW: Psychopathologic precursors and sociodemographic risk factors for the schizophrenia syndrome. Arch Gen Psychiatry 49:37–46, 1992

Vaillant GE: Prospective prediction of schizophrenic remission. Arch Gen Psychiatry 11:509–518, 1964

Van der Velde CD: Variability in schizophrenia: indication of a regulatory disease. Arch Gen Psychiatry 33:489–496, 1976

Van Putten T: The many faces of akathisia. Compr Psychiatry 16:43–47, 1975

Van Putten T, May PR: "Akinetic depression" in schizophrenia. Arch Gen Psychiatry 35:1101–1107, 1978

Villalobos A: A double-blind comparative clinical study of loxapine, diazepam, and placebo in hospitalized patients with various states of anxiety. Current Therapeutics Research 23:243–252, 1978

Williams ME, Hadler NM: Sounding board: the illness as the focus of geriatric medicine. N Engl J Med 308:1357–1360, 1983

Winokur G: Anxiety disorders: relationships to other psychiatric illness. Psychiatr Clin North Am 11:287–293, 1988

Young PC, Labatte LA, Arana GW: Comorbidity of panic disorder and schizophrenia. Poster presentation at the 151st annual meeting of the American Psychiatric Association, Toronto, Ontario, Canada, May 30–June 4, 1998

Yung AR, McGorry PD: The prodromal phase of first episode psychosis: past and current conceptualizations. Schizophr Bull 22:353–370, 1996

Zarate R: The comorbidity between schizophrenia and anxiety disorders. Paper presented to the 31st annual meeting of the Association for the Advancement of Behavior Therapy, Miami Beach, FL, November 13–16, 1997

Zohar J: Is there room for a new diagnostic subtype—the schizoobsessive subtype? CNS Spectrums 2(3):49–50, 1997

Depression in the Course of Schizophrenia

Samuel G. Siris, M.D.

*I*t is generally accepted that the first building block of modern psychiatric nosology was Kraepelin's distinction between those disorders we now know as mood disorders and the illness (or illnesses) we now know as schizophrenia. Nevertheless, beginning with Bleuler (1911/1950), the observation was repeatedly made over the years that a substantial proportion of patients diagnosed with schizophrenia manifest some sort of "depressive-like" symptoms at certain points during their clinical course. These two propositions were difficult to reconcile because the Kraepelinian dichotomy maintained a powerful influence in psychiatry and empirical observations and understanding of the depressive state in patients with schizophrenia were slow to accumulate.

The seeming non sequitur of "depressive" symptoms in schizophrenia, as a consequence of Kraepelin's original observations, generated a tendency either to ignore or to psychologize depressive states in schizophrenia in the early and middle years of the 20th century. In some psychodynamic writings, the question of depression in schizophrenia was written off entirely on the basis of a thesis that schizophrenia patients, by definition, lacked the proper ego structures to develop depression. Elsewhere in the literature, psychodynamic formulations were used to explain states of depression in patients with schizophrenia. Meyer-Gross wrote about depression as being a reaction of despair to the psychotic process and a denial of the future (see McGlashan and Carpenter 1976b). Other central psychodynamic themes included loss (Miller and Sonnenberg 1973; Roth 1970; Semrad 1966) and the notion that a state of depression was a necessary stage in the progression out of the more pathological narcissistic regressed state that was represented by florid psychosis (Semrad 1966). Semrad (1966) also understood the depressed state to be influenced by the pain and/or despair of an "empty ego." Both he and Eissler (1951), however, saw depression in schizophrenia as a moment of therapeutic opportunity, when insight and mastery might overcome more primitive defensive psychotic ego states as they receded. In this light, depression in the course of schizophrenia was seen as a significant positive prognostic sign. Clearly, though, in all these writings, depression tended to be seen not as a diathesis from which the patient was suffering, but rather as a reaction, in one form or another, to the primary illness of schizophrenia and/or its consequences. Little considered was the possibility that a natural diathesis for depression was complicating the course of schizophrenia in any substantial proportion of patients.

In more recent years, however, depression in schizophrenia became the subject of a more data-based approach to research. The frequency and intensity of depression have been documented in patients with schizophrenia (Bowers and Astrachan 1967; McGlashan and Carpenter 1976a; Siris 1991, 2000), as the definitions of both schizophrenia and depression have become more operationalized. In the latter part of the century, with the emergence of psychopharmacology as the central treatment modality for schizophrenia, the prognostic implications of depression appeared to change. Investigators began to observe that the outcomes were less favorable, rather than more favorable, for those schizophrenia patients who manifest depressive symptoms (Falloon et al. 1978). Such patients were noted, then, to be at higher risk for relapse or rehospitalization (Birchwood et al. 1993; Johnson 1988; Mandel et al. 1982; Roy et al. 1983) or even suicide (Caldwell and Gottesman 1990; Drake and Cotton 1986; Roy et al. 1983).

Indeed, it has become recognized, over time, that approximately 10% of schizophrenia patients end their lives in suicide (Caldwell and Gottesman 1990; Miles 1977). Depressive states appear to figure importantly in this, as it has been noted that suicidal ideation is associated with depression in schizophrenia (Barnes et al. 1989) and that many suicides (Drake and Cotton 1986; Heilä et al. 1997; Roy 1982; Stephens et al. 1999) or suicide attempts (Prasad and Kumar 1988; Roy 1986) among persons with schizophrenia involve individuals who have had recent or past histories of depressive symptoms, especially psychological symptoms such as hopelessness (Drake and Cotton 1986). In one study, in fact, more than 80% of the explained variance in suicidal behavior among outpatient schizophrenia patients was accounted for by depression (Bartels et al. 1992).

Over time, a variety of names have been attached to the state of depression occurring in the course of schizophrenia. One of the recurring appellations in the literature is the term *postpsychotic depression,* which, despite the controversy that surrounds it and the confusion it easily engenders with regard to the possibilities of causality, is used in ICD-10 (World Health Organization 1988) and, more recently, in Appendix B of DSM-IV (American Psychiatric Association 1994) to describe this disorder. Much of the confusion about this name stems from the misunderstanding that it implies a depression necessarily occurring immediately after resolution of the psychotic state. This is not the case. Rather, the only implication is that the depressed condition follows the psychosis, but without any specification of the interval—which could be brief, intermediate, or lengthy—as earlier had been clear in the diagnostic category "depression superimposed on residual schizophrenia" included in the Research Diagnostic Criteria (RDC; Spitzer et al. 1978).

But no matter what name is used to describe it, a depression-like syndrome can play a disastrous role in the long-term course of illness in at least some patients with schizophrenia. The syndrome can be associated with substantial reductions in social and vocational functioning and devastating personal suffering for patients and their families. Patients may lose energy, self-esteem, and self-confidence; their ability to concentrate may be impaired; they can lose interest and enjoyment in activities; and sleep, appetite, and motor activities can become dysregulated. Blue mood, pessimism, doubt, guilt, and nihilistic notions may come to dominate the patient's mental life, and it is possible that these themes, and this affect, can become intertwined with the symptoms of the psychosis itself.

Although a variety of hypotheses have been advanced, the etiology and mechanisms of the depressive state in the course of schizophrenia have not been definitively established. Indeed, it is likely that there are a variety of conditions that can mimic a course-related depression in schizophrenia. These range from biological to psychological to social, and from concepts that are an intrinsic component of the schizophrenia diathesis itself to those that are attributable to the environment or extraneous happenstance. An appropriate consideration of the syndrome of depression in the course of schizophrenia, and the approach to its treatment, therefore begin with a consideration of its differential diagnosis.

Differential Diagnosis of Depression in the Course of Schizophrenia

Medical/Organic Factors

A large number of medical/organic factors are possible as causes of depression in patients with schizophrenia (Bartels and Drake 1988). Obviously, any medical/organic factor that can lead to a depressive syndrome in an individual who does not have schizophrenia can also lead to a depressive state in a person with schizophrenia. Such possibilities include a number of common medical conditions (anemia, cancer, neurological disorders, infectious diseases, and metabolic or endocrine disorders), various medications used in the treatment of medical problems (antihypertensive medications such as beta-blockers, sedative-hypnotics, sulfonamides, and indomethacin), and discontinuation of other prescribed medications (most typically corticosteroids and psychostimulants). Substances of abuse, such as alcohol, cannabis, cocaine, and narcotics, can contribute to phenocopies of depression on the basis of acute use, chronic use, or discontinuation. Importantly, the discontinuation of two "legal" substances very commonly used by schizophrenia patients—nicotine and caffeine—can lead to withdrawal states that can mimic depression (Lavin et al. 1996). In particular, "smoke-free" and "decaf" policies on many inpatient units can lead to diagnostic confusion unless the possibility of withdrawal symptoms is considered in the differential diagnosis of "depressive" states.

Negative Symptoms of Schizophrenia

Conceptually, the presentation of negative symptoms in patients with schizophrenia overlaps with the syndrome of depression in a number of domains (Andreasen and Olsen 1982; Bermanzohn and Siris 1992; Carpenter et al. 1985; Crow 1980; Siris et al. 1988a). Overlapping symptoms include poor energy, diminished interest, lack of pleasure, lowered drive state, reduced motor activity, impaired concentration, and general sense of helplessness. Other symptoms, however, may be helpful in making the distinction (Barnes et al. 1989; Kuck et al. 1992; Lindenmayer et al. 1991; Norman and Malla 1991). Blunting of affect, of course, is a feature that is more suggestive of negative symptoms, whereas prominent blue mood, sense of guilt, and suicidal thoughts are more suggestive of depression. Unfortunately, the picture is not always clear, especially since patients with schizophrenia often lack the interpersonal skills and communication abilities necessary to make their own subjective states well known.

Neuroleptic-Induced Dysphoria

Whether neuroleptic medications are "depressogenic" is an unresolved, though hotly debated, issue. Such an effect might be expected, on a theoretical basis, because dopamine synapses are involved in the brain pathways that medicate "reward" (Harrow et al. 1994; Wise 1982). Blocking of pleasure or reward by dopamine blockade, therefore, possibly could lead to anhedonia and a generalized state of depression. Indeed, one well-designed study found more anhedonia and depression in schizophrenia patients who were taking neuroleptics in the maintenance phase of treatment than in those who were not (Harrow et al. 1994). This study built on a series of earlier, more anecdotal reports that implicated neuroleptics in the etiology of depression among schizophrenia patients (DeAlarcon and Carney 1969; Floru et al. 1975; Galdi 1983; Galdi et al. 1981; Johnson 1981a).

The bulk of the controlled-study evidence, however, has tended to refute the proposition that appropriate doses of neuroleptic medication lead to the development of depressive states in individuals with schizophrenia (Knights and Hirsch 1981; Moller and von Zerssen 1986; Siris 1991, 2000). Three types of studies have been involved in this negative evidence. The first involved assessment of schizophrenia patients during the course of their treatment for acute episodes of psychosis. When the appropriate questions were asked, it was ascertained that the greatest levels of depressive symptoms corresponded to the times when the patients were most psychotic and that the symptoms tended to resolve, albeit sometimes at a slower rate, when the psychotic episode was treated with neuroleptic medication (Green et al. 1990; Hirsch et al. 1989; Knights and Hirsch 1981; Leff et al. 1988; Moller and von Zerssen 1982; Strian et al. 1982; Szymanski et al. 1983). These observations therefore suggest that depressive symptoms that were present before the neuroleptic was administered actually decreased during the course of neuroleptic treatment. The second group of studies comprised those that compared the ongoing course of schizophrenia in patients who were treated with neuroleptic medications with the course in those who did not receive such treatment. The patients treated with neuroleptics were not found to demonstrate more depression (Hirsch et al. 1973, 1989; Hogarty and Munetz 1984; Wistedt and Palmstierna 1983). The third group of studies involved comparisons of schizophrenia patients with and without depression, which failed to show any differences in neuroleptic doses or neuroleptic blood levels between the groups (Bandelow et al. 1991; Barnes et al. 1989; Berrios and Bulbena 1987; Roy 1984; Roy et al. 1983; Siris et al. 1988b).

Finally, relevant to this issue, one popular hypothesis concerning the pathophysiology of schizophrenia is that schizophrenia represents a disorder of dopamine regulation (Davis et al. 1991). Simply put, this conceptualization posits schizophrenia patients as being "brittle" in terms of their dopamine regulation—that is, being vulnerable to the occurrence of dopamine storms (psychosis) and dopamine droughts (negative symptoms). Within this framework it is easy to imagine how the administration of more than the minimum required amount of neuroleptic (dopamine-blocking) medication during relatively psychosis-free intervals could exacerbate negative symptoms, which, in turn, because they can present a close phenocopy of depression as noted earlier, can give the impression of neuroleptic-induced depression.

Neuroleptic-Induced Akinesia

The extrapyramidal side effect of neuroleptic-induced akinesia has had more than one definition in the literature, and this can be a confusing point. The original definition, and the one that is easiest to recognize, involves stiffness with cogwheel rigidity of large muscle groups, leading to typical parkinsonian posture, shuffling gait, and reduction of accessory motor movements (Chien et al. 1984). These symptoms are gross, and the diagnosis of this type of akinesia is relatively easy.

A later definition, originally formulated by Rifkin et al. (1975, 1978) and elaborated by Van Putten and May (1978), is more subtle but describes an equally debilitating condition (Bermanzohn and Siris 1992; Martin et al. 1985). This form of akinesia, also extrapyramidal in origin, involves a reduction in the basal ganglia's ability to initiate and sustain behavior. Patients with this form of akinesia may or may not have decreased accessory motor movements, but behaviorally they are "like bumps on a log" and act as if "their starter motor is broken." If they are watching television, for example, they are likely not to get up spontaneously and do something else at the end of the show they are watching. Rather, they are likely to "just sit." In fact, if the condition is severe, they are likely not to even have the spontaneity to change the channel to find a show they like. They also appear to lack initiative socially—a problem that may be manifested by a lack of ordinary interpersonal behaviors such as starting conversations in appropriate situations. Blue mood has also been noted to accompany this state. Obviously, when asked about their condition, patients with this form of akinesia are likely to report anhedonia, self-blame, and the subjective state of lack of energy (a state easily confused with depression). Indeed, it is unfortunate that a large proportion of the studies that have examined the incidence or treatment of depression in patients with schizophrenia have not appropriately considered the possibility of this form of akinesia as a confounding factor and controlled for it either by a reduction in neuroleptic dose or by concomitant administration of full doses of antiparkinsonian medications.

Neuroleptic-Induced Akathisia

A second extrapyramidal neuroleptic side effect that is easy to diagnose in its blatant form but that in its more subtle form can easily be confused with depression is *akathisia* (Siris 1985; Van Putten 1975). In akathisia, it is "as if the patient's starter motor won't shut off." Prominent motor restlessness makes the blatant form of this side effect obvious. Subtle forms can be more difficult to recognize, manifesting as a more modest propensity for increased motor behavior, perhaps some degree of wandering or over-talkativeness, or more excessive behavioral responses in situations than otherwise would occur. In some patients, this can appear to be agitation. Importantly, akathisia is often experienced by patients as substantially dysphoric (Halstead et al. 1994; Van Putten 1975), and, indeed, akathisia has been associated with both suicidal ideation and suicidal behavior (Drake and Ehrlich 1985; Shear et al. 1983). Like akinesia, akathisia is likely to respond to a lowering of the neuroleptic dosage, if that can be achieved. Akathisia is less likely to respond to antiparkinsonian medication, however, although it may respond to benzodiazepines or beta-blockers (Fleisch-haker et al. 1990).

Disappointment Reactions

People with schizophrenia may easily have as much, if not more, to be disappointed about in the way in which their lives are progressing as individuals who do not have schizophrenia, and their interpersonal or communication difficulties may make it more difficult than it otherwise would be to distinguish this situation from depression at any given point in time. Acute disappointment reactions can be distinguished by the parallel history of a suitable recent event (if that can be elicited) and a transient course (seldom more than a few days to a couple weeks). Chronic disappointment reactions are known as *demoralization* (de Figueiredo 1993; Frank 1973; Klein 1974) and can be more difficult to distinguish from depression. A chronic history of disappointment or failure can lead a person with schizophrenia to the conviction that a useful or satisfying life is impossible. Indeed, it has been empirically validated that schizophrenia patients who feel less of a sense of control regarding their illness are more likely to experience depression (Birchwood et al. 1993). Of course, it is also reasonable to believe that the demoralization state is worthy of diagnosis and understanding because it is particularly likely to be amenable to appropriate psychosocial interventions.

Prodrome of Psychotic Relapse

Studies that have reviewed or examined the process of decompensation into psychotic episodes in schizophrenia often have noted symptoms common to depression to be manifest at these times (Docherty et al. 1978;

Green et al. 1990; Herz 1985; Herz and Melville 1980; Hirsch et al. 1989; Johnson 1988; Tollefson et al. 1999). Anxiety and withdrawal are frequent accompaniments of dysphoria in this situation, and signs or symptoms of early psychotic decompensation, such as hypervigilance or overinterpretation of events, may provide a valuable clue as to the true nature of the psychotic prodrome. Usually the depressed-appearing state is short-lived when it is a component of the psychotic prodrome, lasting for a couple days to a week, before more prominent and definitive symptoms of psychosis become manifest.

Schizoaffective Depression

Conceptually, the diagnosis of schizoaffective disorder pertains when the patient's presentation of the full depressive syndrome coincides with the florid psychotic syndrome in patients who also have been psychotic in the absence of an affective syndrome. This situation has been defined differently according to various diagnostic schemes (Coryell et al. 1990; Levitt and Tsuang 1988; Taylor 1992), the application of which can cause some variation in the exact boundary between "depression in schizophrenia" and "schizoaffective depression." The diagnosis of schizoaffective disorder opens up a set of treatment options that may be valuable but that take us beyond the scope of the present chapter (Siris 1996; Siris and Lavin 1995). The issue of schizoaffective disorder, of course, also enters into the consideration of postpsychotic depression in schizophrenia, because postpsychotic depression occurs in schizoaffective disorder as well. There have been no specific studies of the latter situation; clinical trials have essentially collapsed the latter group of patients with the former under the assumption that the same interventions are applicable in these two circumstances.

Depression as the Expression of a Biological Diathesis in the Course of Schizophrenia

Finally, after the other elements of the differential diagnosis noted earlier in this section have been ruled out, we are left with the possibility of a depression based on a biological diathesis occurring in an individual otherwise correctly diagnosed with schizophrenia. The determination of this issue, at least at the present time, is inexact, since there is no available direct biological way to ascertain the presence of a biological diathesis for depression—or, for that matter, schizophrenia. Specifically, there is no biopsy, electrical test, chemical test, radiological test, genetic marker, or even autopsy finding that can definitively establish such a psychiatric diagnosis. Instead, we are limited to phenomenological descriptors and patients' own accounts of their subjective states in arriving at our diagnoses.

Indeed, patients' responses to medications have frequently been used historically as validators for the symptom lists we have come to employ today to establish the boundaries of diagnoses such as depression and schizophrenia—a use of "predicate logic" that clinicians would readily recognize as flawed if they saw a patient using it to arrive at an important conclusion. On the other hand, since clinicians are fundamentally interested in identifying the most sensible treatment for suffering dysfunctional individuals when they employ a diagnostic scheme, this approach has validity in that appropriate treatments may be suggested even if the logic might be flawed and the underlying biological assumptions might not be correct. The discussion of treatment issues that occurs later in this chapter certainly should be interpreted with this in mind.

Incidence and Prevalence of Depression in Patients With Schizophrenia

More than two dozen studies have been published examining the rates of occurrence of depression in the course of schizophrenia (Koreen et al. 1993; Sands and Harrow 1999; Siris 1991, 1995; Tapp et al. 1994). They have varied considerably in terms of a number of methodological considerations: the definition employed for schizophrenia, the definition used for depression, the interval surveyed, the methodology of the survey, and the patients' treatment status at the time of the observation. The most notable conclusion that can be drawn from these studies is that, no matter what definitions and conditions prevail, at least some meaningful rate of phenotypic depression is observed in the course of schizophrenia.

Among these studies, the rates of depression varied from a low of 7% in a cross-sectional assessment of patients with DSM-III-defined schizophrenia who were chronically hospitalized and in whom an effort was made to distinguish depression from negative symptoms (Hirsch et al. 1989), to a high of 75% for at least one positive assessment of depression by either one of two criteria among patients with "first break" RDC-defined schizophrenia who were evaluated on a weekly to monthly basis for up to 5 years (Koreen et al. 1993). The modal rate for all these studies was 25%, a fair benchmark that has endured through the course of a number of reviews (Johnson 1981b; Mandel et al. 1982; McGlashan and Carpenter 1976b; Siris 1991, 1995; Winokur 1972).

Since depression is observed more frequently in females among people without schizophrenia (Kessler et al. 1993), and since the expression of schizophrenia in general is different in women than it is in men in a number of ways (Goldstein and Link 1988), it would be interesting to know if sex differences are observed with regard to the presentation of depression in patients with schizophrenia (Goldstein and Tsuang 1990; Seeman 1997). Indeed, such differences, if found, would have theoretical nosological implications (Goldstein et al. 1990; Seeman 1996b). Unfortunately, in most studies sex has not been specifically examined with reference to depression in schizophrenia, especially in any way that attempts to account for the various elements of the differential diagnosis outlined earlier. Addington et al. (1996), in the strongest attempt to rule out negative symptoms and extrapyramidal side effects in a prospective assessment of depression with the Calgary Depression Scale for Schizophrenia, found similar rates of depression for both sexes. Several other studies also failed to find significant differences between the sexes in terms of depression rates in patients with schizophrenia (Haas et al. 1990; Hafner et al. 1994; Shtasel et al. 1992). On the other hand, three careful chart reviews have suggested such differences: McGlashan and Bardenstein (1990) examined Chestnut Lodge patients according to a dichotomous variable (depressed vs. not depressed) and found that women with schizophrenia were more likely to be depressed than men with schizophrenia; Goldstein et al. (1990), also using a dichotomous variable, found more dysphoria (not exactly the same as "depression") in females with schizophrenia (54%) than in males with schizophrenia (45%) in the Iowa-500 and Iowa non-500 data; and Goldstein and Link (1988) found female schizophrenia inpatients to have more depressed mood than male schizophrenia inpatients. In this last study, the investigators also found a relationship between depressed mood and psychosis in women with schizophrenia but not in men with schizophrenia. Other data suggest that negative symptoms may be more depression-like in women with schizophrenia than they are in men with schizophrenia (Lewine 1985).

Additionally, with regard to sex differences, it is relevant to note that women's psychopathology ratings worsen in general during that phase of the menstrual cycle when estrogen levels are low (Hallonquist et al. 1993; Riecher-Rossler et al. 1994; Seeman 1996a, 1997), and that this is likely to be true for depression ratings. However, depressed mood may not always be exacerbated by low estrogen levels (Hafner et al. 1994), and this effect is certainly not specific to schizophrenia. Results from large-scale, controlled prospective studies of focusing on the symptom of depression in female schizophrenia patients over the course of the menstrual cycle have not been published. Thus, overall, although it is likely that there might be some differences in the rates or expression of depression in women and men with schizophrenia, this phenomenology has not yet been fully clarified with prospective observations.

Treatment Strategies

An appropriate treatment approach to depression begins with a consideration of the differential diagnostic possibilities outlined earlier in this chapter. Obviously, since there are no available biological tests (except for the medical/organic conditions), or even psychological tests, that are known to be informative in drawing these diagnostic distinctions, these diagnoses must be made on a purely clinical basis. Since an acute transient disappointment reaction and a prodrome of a new psychotic episode are both possibilities when a new episode of depression appears in the course of schizophrenia, the prudent course is to react to such a new episode with increased frequency of surveillance. If the episode is a transient disappointment reaction, it will soon resolve spontaneously, and no other intervention beyond nonspecific support is indicated. However, if the new onset of depression is the first harbinger of a new episode of psychosis, increased surveillance will allow this new episode to be caught quickly and "nipped in the bud" as much as possible through appropriate antipsychotic interventions.

For a neuroleptic-treated schizophrenia patient with a continuing episode of depression, the next consideration is whether the neuroleptic medication is contributing to the manifestations of depression. This could occur on the basis of either the hypothesized neuroleptic-induced dysphoria state or the extrapyramidal side effects of akinesia or akathisia. A reduction of neuroleptic dosage would be the first choice of how to treat any of these conditions, if there is leeway to accomplish that safely. A trial of a so-called atypical antipsychotic agent also may be quite helpful in this situation. Otherwise, a full dose of an antiparkinsonian medication, built up in suitable gradations, is the treatment of choice for the possibility of neuroleptic-induced akinesia. If the depressive syndrome is thought to be the product of akathisia and an antiparkinsonian medication trial proves not to be helpful, a benzodiazepine or beta-blocker trial can be attempted.

After a transient disappointment reaction, prodrome of psychosis, and neuroleptic side effect have been eliminated, as best as possible, as the cause of a continuing state of postpsychotic depression in schizophrenia, a trial of treatment with an antidepressant medication should be considered as an adjunct to the patient's antipsychotic (and perhaps antiparkinsonian drug) regimen. Table 2–1 shows the detailed results of the double-blind, controlled studies that have examined this approach. Although the results are mixed, the studies that are methodologically the strongest are the ones that most support the efficacy and safety of an adjunctive antidepressant trial in this situation (Plasky 1991; Siris 1991, 1995, 2000). More

Table 2–1. Double-blind studies of antidepressants in "depressed" schizophrenia patients

Study	N	Sample/Study characteristics	Neuroleptic	Antidepressant	Duration	Result(s)
Singh et al. 1978	60	Chronic inpatients with symptoms of depression Schizophrenia defined by Feighner criteria Ham-D score of 18 or more	Previous phenothiazine continued	Trazodone 300 mg/day or placebo	6 wk	More favorable response with trazodone, as measured by Ham-D and CGI changes No significant differences in BPRS scores
Prusoff et al. 1979	35	Outpatients Schizophrenia defined by New Haven Index criteria Score of at least 7 on the RDRS	Perphenazine 16–48 mg/day	Amitriptyline 100–200 mg/day or placebo	1, 2, 4, or 6 mo	With amitriptyline: Some decrease in depression ratings Some increase in thought disorder and agitation ratings Improvement in social well-being Overall impression: mildly positive response
Waehrens and Gerlach 1980	17	"Long-term" inpatients Cross-over design "Schizophrenia" (no criteria given) Chronic and "emotionally withdrawn"	Continuation of previous neuroleptics	Maprotiline 50–200 mg/day or placebo	8 wk	No benefit found from addition of maprotiline

Table 2–1. Double-blind studies of antidepressants in "depressed" schizophrenia patients (continued)

Study	N	Sample/Study characteristics	Neuroleptic	Antidepressant	Duration	Result(s)
Johnson 1981a	50	All "chronic" patients (unstated if inpatients or outpatients) Schizophrenia defined by Feighner or Schneiderian symptoms BDI score of 15 or more for episode of "acute" depression	Fluphenazine decanoate or flupenthixol decanoate (doses not specified)	Nortriptyline 150 mg/day or placebo	5 wk	No statistically significant benefit to depression from addition of nortriptyline, though 40% placebo response rate would make such a finding difficult to detect Increased side effects with nortriptyline
Kurland and Nagaraju 1981	22	Inpatients Schizophrenia (no criteria given) Ham-D score of 18 or more Patients treated with antiparkinsonian medications were specifically excluded	Chlorpromazine 75–300 mg/day or haloperidol 6–15 mg/day	Viloxazine up to 300 mg/day maximum in final week only or placebo	4 wk	No differences between groups Majority of patients in both groups improved
Becker 1983	52	Inpatients Schizophrenia defined by RDC Major depressive syndrome (superimposed on schizophrenia) defined by RDC	Chlorpromazine 100–1,200 mg/day or thiothixene 5–60 mg/day	Imipramine 150–250 mg/day for patients on chlorpromazine, or placebo for patients on thiothixene	4 wk[a]	Both treatments effective compared with baseline on BPRS and Ham-D, but neither treatment statistically superior to the other More sedative and autonomic side effects with chlorpromazine-imipramine combination

Table 2–1. Double-blind studies of antidepressants in "depressed" schizophrenia patients (*continued*)

Study	N	Sample/Study characteristics	Neuroleptic	Antidepressant	Duration	Result(s)
Siris et al. 1987	33	Outpatients Schizophrenia or schizoaffective disorder defined by RDC (nonpsychotic or residually psychotic) Major or minor depression defined by RDC Depression unresponsive to benztropine 2 mg po tid	Fluphenazine decanoate (clinically adjusted stable weekly dose)	Imipramine 150–200 mg/day or placebo	6 wk	Imipramine group superior on global measure (CGI) and depression scales No difference between groups in psychosis or side effects
Dufresne et al. 1988	38	Inpatients Schizophrenia defined by DSM-III Superimposed atypical affective disorder (equivalent to DSM-III major depression)	Thiothixene (clinically adjusted stable dose)	Bupropion 150–750 mg/day flexible dose or placebo	4 wk	Both groups improved, but placebo group improved more Majority of bupropion-treated patients dropped out
Kramer et al. 1989	58	Inpatients, actively psychotic Initial DSM-III diagnosis of schizophrenia Schizoaffective disorder (mainly schizophrenic), depressive subtype defined by RDC Ham-D score of more than 17 Treated with benztropine 2–8 mg/day	Haloperidol 0.4 mg/kg/day po	Amitriptyline 3.5 mg/kg/day, desipramine 3.5 mg/kg/day, or placebo	4 wk	Neither addition of amitriptyline nor addition of desipramine showed significant therapeutic advantage Patients treated with an antidepressant tended to score worse at the end on BPRS hallucinatory behavior and thinking disturbance

Table 2–1. Double-blind studies of antidepressants in "depressed" schizophrenia patients (continued)

Study	N	Sample/Study characteristics	Neuroleptic	Antidepressant	Duration	Result(s)
Siris et al. 1994	24	Outpatients Schizophrenia or schizoaffective disorder defined by RDC (nonpsychotic or residually psychotic) Major depression defined by RDC History of favorable response to adjunctive imipramine (150–300 mg/day)	Fluphenazine decanoate (clinically adjusted stable dose)	Open continuation treatment with imipramine 100–300 mg/day for 6 months Then imipramine either maintained or tapered to placebo, double-blind for 1-year maintenance trial	18 mo	Significantly more relapse into depression in group whose antidepressant was tapered to placebo No exacerbation of psychosis while patients receiving adjunctive imipramine, and significantly more exacerbation of psychosis in group whose antidepressant was tapered to placebo

Note. BDI = Beck Depression Inventory; BPRS = Brief Psychiatric Rating Scale; CGI = Clinical Global Impression; Ham-D = Hamilton Rating Scale for Depression; RDRS = Raskin Depression Rating Scale.
[a]After 2 weeks drug free.
Source. Adapted from Siris 1991.

favorable results were found among outpatients than among inpatients (Fisher exact test, $P = 0.048$ for the studies in Table 2–1), and less favorable results seemed to be obtained among patients who were prominently psychotic at the time of the adjunctive antidepressant trial (Kramer et al. 1989) than among those who were not psychotic at the time of the trial. Only one study has been reported concerning the efficacy of maintenance adjunctive antidepressant medication for patients who appeared to respond favorably initially (Siris et al. 1994). That study indicated that indefinite maintenance medication appeared to be warranted among patients who initially had responded favorably. Interestingly, patients receiving maintenance adjunctive antidepressant medication experienced fewer relapses into depression ($P = 0.0007$) and fewer exacerbations of psychosis ($P = 0.018$) than did those receiving maintenance adjunctive placebo. Half of the relapses into depression in the control group were accompanied by increases in psychosis ratings; none of the patients maintained on adjunctive antidepressant medication experienced such increases. This raises the possibility that preventing a relapse into depression may be associated with patients' not entering a concurrent exacerbation of psychosis. It also suggests that maintenance of adjunctive antidepressant medication may have been protective in this regard.

As shown in Table 2–1, the studies of antidepressants in treating postpsychotic depression in patients with schizophrenia generally have involved cyclic antidepressants. Selective serotonin reuptake inhibitors (SSRIs) and monoamine oxidase inhibitors (MAOIs) have not been adequately tested for this condition, although anecdotal information suggests that they may be useful. However, there have been encouraging double-blind trials of SSRIs (Goff et al. 1995; Silver and Nassar 1992; Spina et al. 1994) and MAOIs (Bodkin et al. 1996; Bucci 1987; Perenyi et al. 1992) for "negative symptoms" in schizophrenia.

It is also possible that there may be a role for the use of lithium in at least some cases of depression in patients with schizophrenia, although, again, proper studies of this issue have not been reported. Most reports involving lithium in the treatment of patients with schizophrenia have examined its acute use in psychotic exacerbations rather than during the maintenance phase of treatment (Christison et al. 1991; Plasky 1991), with the most frequently cited indicators of favorable response being excitement, overactivity, and euphoria rather than depression. Nevertheless, depressive symptoms have occasionally been identified as a favorable prognosticator of adjunctive lithium response in patients with schizophrenia (Lerner et al. 1988), in addition to previous affective episodes, a family history of affective illness, and an overall episodic course (Atre-Vaidya and Taylor 1989).

A discussion of treatment strategies for depression in patients with schizophrenia is not complete without consideration of psychosocial interventions, even though controlled studies of these modalities have not been carried out in a specifically depressed schizophrenia patient population. Appropriate psychosocial modalities certainly can be valuable in the long-term management of schizophrenia (Hogarty et al. 1986). These approaches include stress reduction strategies, psychoeducation, skill building, instruction in problem-solving techniques, and family interventions targeted to minimizing expressed emotion. Interventions aimed at enhancing hope and self-esteem also may be useful.

Vulnerability, Stress, and Psychiatric Diatheses: A Hypothetical Model

Figure 2–1 depicts an integrative schema that conceptualizes the interplay of extrinsic and intrinsic factors with the schizophrenia diathesis. The basis for this formulation is the familiar stress-diathesis model of schizophrenia (Nuechterlein and Dawson 1984; Zubin and Spring 1977), supported by more recent understanding of the neuropsychological underpinnings of the pathophysiology of schizophrenia (Weinberger 1987).

In Figure 2–1, the vertical axis represents vulnerability to psychotic symptoms of the schizophrenic type and the horizontal axis depicts the proportion of the general population. At the far left, a tiny fraction of the population manifests a very high vulnerability to psychosis, with an ever-decreasing loading for such risk moving to the right along the curve. Only a fraction of 1% of the population express a vulnerability so great that a schizophrenic psychosis will emerge under virtually any level of life stress, no matter how minor. However, several percent of the population have a meaningful but lesser degree of vulnerability, such that the schizophrenic psychosis will become manifest if a great enough stress is encountered to "push the patient over the brink." This stress can come from any of a variety of sources and can be biological, psychological, or social.

The model depicted fits much of what we know about schizophrenia and what can influence its expression. If the fundamental vulnerability is genetic, additional biopsychosocial stressors might be poor maternal nutrition (associated with poverty), intrauterine viral infection, injuries during a difficult delivery, inadequate childhood nutrition, lack of normal childhood stimulation, lack of opportunity to learn protective interpersonal and coping skills, developmental experiences promoting intrapsychic conflicts, extreme psychic stress in adolescence/early adulthood (e.g.,

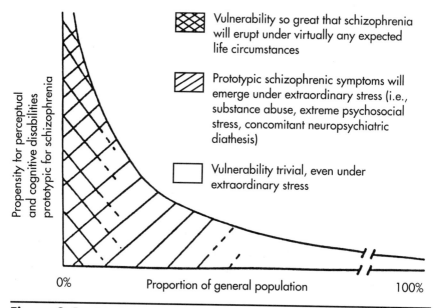

Figure 2–1. Model of vulnerability, stress, and schizophrenic diathesis. Integrative schema conceptualizing the interplay of extrinsic and intrinsic factors with the schizophrenic diathesis.

Source. Reprinted with permission from Siris SG, Lavin MR: "Schizoaffective Disorder, Schizophreniform Disorder and Acute Psychotic Disorder (Including Brief Reactive Psychosis)," in *Comprehensive Textbook of Psychiatry/VI*, 6th Edition. Edited by Kaplan HI, Sadock BJ. Philadelphia, PA, Williams & Wilkins, 1995, pp. 1019–1031 (p. 1021). Copyright 1995, Williams & Wilkins.

high "expressed emotion," poverty, trauma, chaotic environments), and the biological, psychological, and social insults that may be associated with substance use and abuse. Once the patient is "pushed over the brink" into psychosis, of course, the full physiological and biopsychosocial cascade of events is unleashed, representing the multivariate clinical course of schizophrenia.

A novel integrative model posits that the diathesis for an independent psychiatric disorder may represent the stressor that can tip a person with an intermediate vulnerability over into the path of psychotic deterioration (Siris 1988; Siris and Lavin 1995). Thus, a person who has a diathesis for a major depressive disorder accompanying his or her intermediate diathesis for schizophrenia could be tipped over by the stress of the affective disorder into a schizophrenic psychosis. Certainly, a person with depression is sorely stressed psychologically. It is not unreasonable to speculate that such a person is stressed biologically and socially as well.

Since, as depicted in Figure 2–1, there are many more people with intermediate vulnerabilities to the schizophrenic psychosis than with extreme vulnerability, the chances of a psychosis being triggered by another concurrent psychiatric diathesis can be considerable. For example, if this proposed model were the basis for so-called schizoaffective disorder, it could account for schizoaffective disorder being roughly as prevalent as schizophrenia in the general population (Siris and Lavin 1995). This model, of course, also opens the possibility that other concurrent psychiatric diatheses, such as those for panic disorder or obsessive-compulsive disorder, could interact with an intermediate vulnerability for psychosis in a similar manner.

Several of the issues discussed earlier are consistent with this model involving depression in schizophrenia. One is the observation that depressive-like symptoms are a common component of the psychotic prodrome (Docherty et al. 1978; Green et al. 1990; Herz 1985; Herz and Melville 1980; Hirsch et al. 1989; Johnson 1988; Tollefson et al. 1999). Dysphoria also has been found to be more strongly associated with positive symptoms in schizophrenia than with negative symptoms (Norman and Malla 1994). However, since simple dysthymia is not overrepresented in patients with schizophrenia the way depression is (Bland et al. 1987), the role of depression in schizophrenia cannot readily be accounted for as a mere psychological reaction to the unfolding of unpleasant events. Also relevant is the finding that maintenance adjunctive antidepressant treatment in responding postpsychotic depressed patients protected them not only from relapses into depression but from psychotic exacerbations as well (Siris et al. 1994).

Although the model proposed here is by no means proven, it is rich in testable hypotheses and possibly could account for a portion of the heterogeneity well known to be a component of the disorder we refer to as schizophrenia. Additionally, and importantly, it is a model with implications for treatment, to relieve suffering and promote functioning among a substantial number of patients afflicted with symptoms of both schizophrenia and depression.

In summary, it is well described that a depressive syndrome often occurs in the course of schizophrenia. However, this syndrome is not homogeneous. Rather, there is a broad differential diagnosis that is crucial both for our understanding of its etiology in any specific case and for our arriving at a rational approach to its treatment. Moreover, the occurrence of a depressive syndrome in the course of schizophrenia raises theoretical issues relevant to the interplay of psychosis with both situational events and affective diatheses in psychiatry. These are issues that cut to the very core of our understanding of the disorder we know as schizophrenia, suggesting novel approaches to the organization of its heterogeneity as well as testable hypotheses concerning a variety of therapeutic interventions.

References

Addington D, Addington J, Patten S: Gender and affect in schizophrenia. Can J Psychiatry 41:265–268, 1996

American Psychiatric Association: Diagnostic and Statistical Manual of Mental Disorders. Washington, DC, American Psychiatric Association, 1994

Andreasen NC, Olsen S: Negative vs positive schizophrenia: definition and validation. Arch Gen Psychiatry 39:789–794, 1982

Atre-Vaidya N, Taylor MA: Effectiveness of lithium in schizophrenia: do we really have an answer? J Clin Psychiatry 50:170–173, 1989

Bandelow B, Muller P, Gaebel WE: Depressive syndromes in schizophrenic patients after discharge from hospital. Eur Arch Psychiatry Clin Neurosci 240:113–120, 1991

Barnes TR, Curson DA, Liddle PF, et al: The nature and prevalence of depression in chronic schizophrenic in-patients. Br J Psychiatry 154:486–491, 1989

Bartels SJ, Drake RE: Depressive symptoms in schizophrenia: comprehensive differential diagnosis. Compr Psychiatry 29:467–483, 1988

Bartels SJ, Drake RE, McHugo GJ: Alcohol abuse, depression and suicidal behavior in schizophrenia. Am J Psychiatry 149:394–395, 1992

Becker RE: Implications of the efficacy of thiothixene and a chlorpromazine-imipramine combination for depression in schizophrenia. Am J Psychiatry 140:208–211, 1983

Bermanzohn PC, Siris SG: Akinesia: A syndrome common to parkinsonism, retarded depression, and negative symptoms. Compr Psychiatry 33:221–232, 1992

Berrios GE, Bulbena A: Post psychotic depression: the Fulbourn cohort. Acta Psychiatr Scand 76:89–93, 1987

Birchwood M, Mason R, Macmillan F, et al: Depression, demoralization and control over psychotic illness: a comparison of depressed and non-depressed patients with a chronic psychosis. Psychol Med 23:387–395, 1993

Bland RC, Newman SC, Orn H: Schizophrenia: lifetime co-morbidity in a community sample. Acta Psychiatr Scand 75:383–391, 1987

Bleuler E: Dementia Praecox, or the Group of Schizophrenias (1911). New York, International Universities Press, 1950

Bodkin AJ, Cohen BM, Salomon MS, et al: Treatment of negative symptoms in schizophrenia and schizoaffective disorder by selegiline augmentation of antipsychotic medication. J Nerv Ment Dis 184:295–301, 1996

Bowers MD, Astrachan BM: Depression in acute schizophrenia. Am J Psychiatry 123:976–979, 1967

Bucci L: The negative symptoms of schizophrenia and the monoamine oxidase inhibitors. Psychopharmacology (Berl) 91:104–108, 1987

Caldwell CB, Gottesman II: Schizophrenics kill themselves too: a review of risk factors for suicide. Schizophr Bull 16:571–589, 1990

Carpenter WT Jr, Heinrichs DW, Alphs LD: Treatment of negative symptoms. Schizophr Bull 11:440–452, 1985

Chien CP, DiMascio A, Cole JD: Antiparkinson agents and depot phenothiazines. Am J Psychiatry 131:86–90, 1984

Christison GW, Kirch DG, Wyatt RJ: When symptoms persist: choosing among alternative somatic treatments for schizophrenia. Schizophr Bull 17:217–240, 1991

Coryell W, Keller M, Lavori P, et al: Affective syndromes, psychotic features, and prognosis, I: depression. Arch Gen Psychiatry 47:651–657, 1990

Crow TJ: Molecular pathology of schizophrenia: more than one disease process? BMJ 280:66–68, 1980

Davis KL, Kahn RS, Ko G, et al: Dopamine in schizophrenia: a review and reconceptualization. Am J Psychiatry 148:1474–1486, 1991

DeAlarcon R, Carney MWP: Severe depressive mood changes following slow-release intramuscular fluphenazine injection. BMJ 3:564–567, 1969

de Figueiredo JM: Depression and demoralization: phenomenologic differences and research perspectives. Compr Psychiatry 34:308–311, 1993

Docherty JP, van Kammen DP, Siris SG, et al: Stages of onset of acute schizophrenic psychosis. Am J Psychiatry 135:720–726, 1978

Drake RE, Cotton PG: Depression, hopelessness and suicide in chronic schizophrenia. Br J Psychiatry 148:554–559, 1986

Drake RE, Ehrlich J: Suicide attempts associated with akathisia. Am J Psychiatry 142:499–501, 1985

Dufresne RL, Kass DJ, Becker RE: Buproprion and thiothixene versus placebo and thiothixene in the treatment of depression in schizophrenia. Drug Development Research 12:259–266, 1988

Eissler KR: Remarks on the psycho-analysis of schizophrenia. Int J Psychoanal 32:139–156, 1951

Falloon I, Watt DC, Shepherd M: A comparative controlled trial of pimozide and fluphenazine decanoate in the continuation therapy of schizophrenia. Psychol Med 8:59–70, 1978

Fleischhaker WW, Roth SD, Kane JM: The pharmacologic treatment of neuroleptic-induced akathisia. J Clin Psychopharmacol 10:12–21, 1990

Floru L, Heinrich K, Wittek F: The problem of post-psychotic schizophrenic depressions and their pharmacological induction. International Pharmacopsychiatry 10:230–239, 1975

Frank JD: Persuasion and Healing. Baltimore, MD, Johns Hopkins University Press, 1973

Galdi J: The causality of depression in schizophrenia. Br J Psychiatry 142:621–625, 1983

Galdi J, Rieder RO, Silber D, et al: Genetic factors in the response to neuroleptics in schizophrenia: a pharmacogenetic study. Psychol Med 11:713–728, 1981

Goff DC, Midha KK, Sarid-Segal O, et al: A placebo-controlled trial of fluoxetine added to neuroleptic in patients with schizophrenia. Psychopharmacology (Berl) 117:417–423, 1995

Goldstein JM, Link BG: Gender and the expression of schizophrenia. J Psychiatr Res 22:141–155, 1988

Goldstein JM, Tsuang MT: Gender and schizophrenia: an introduction and synthesis of findings. Schizophr Bull 16:179–183, 1990

Goldstein JM, Santangelo SL, Simpson JC, et al: The role of gender in identifying subtypes of schizophrenia: a latent class analytic approach. Schizophr Bull 16:263–275, 1990

Green MF, Nuechterlein KH, Ventura J, et al: The temporal relationship between depressive and psychotic symptoms in recent-onset schizophrenia. Am J Psychiatry 147:179–182, 1990

Haas GL, Glick ID, Clarkin JF, et al: Gender and schizophrenia outcome: a clinical trial of an inpatient family intervention. Schizophr Bull 16:277–292, 1990

Hafner H, Maurer K, Loffler W, et al: The epidemiology of early schizophrenia: influence of age and gender on onset and early course. Br J Psychiatry 164 (suppl 23):29–38, 1994

Hallonquist JD, Seeman MV, Lang M, et al: Variation in symptom severity over the menstrual cycle of schizophrenics. Biol Psychiatry 33:207–209, 1993

Halstead SM, Barnes TRE, Speller JC: Akathisia: prevalence and associated dysphoria in an in-patient population with chronic schizophrenia. Br J Psychiatry 164:177–183, 1994

Harrow M, Yonan CA, Sands JR, et al: Depression in schizophrenia: are neuroleptics, akinesia, or anhedonia involved? Schizophr Bull 20:327–338, 1994

Heilä H, Isometsä ET, Henriksson MM, et al: A nationwide psychological autopsy study on age- and sex-specific clinical characteristics of 92 suicide victims with schizophrenia. Am J Psychiatry 154:1235–1242, 1997

Herz M: Prodromal symptoms and prevention of relapse in schizophrenia. J Clin Psychiatry 46 (no 11, sec 2):22–25, 1985

Herz M, Melville C: Relapse in schizophrenia. Am J Psychiatry 137:801–805, 1980

Hirsch SR, Gaind R, Rohde PD, et al: Outpatient maintenance of chronic schizophrenic patients with long-acting fluphenazine: double-blind placebo trial. BMJ 1(854):633–637, 1973

Hirsch SR, Jolley AG, Barnes TRE, et al: Dysphoric and depressive symptoms in chronic schizophrenia. Schizophr Res 2:259–264, 1989

Hogarty GE, Munetz MR: Pharmacogenic depression among outpatient schizophrenic patients: a failure to substantiate. J Clin Psychopharmacol 4:17–24, 1984

Hogarty GE, Anderson CM, Reiss DJ, et al: Family psychoeducational, social skills training, and maintenance chemotherapy in the aftercare treatment of schizophrenia, 1: one-year effects of a controlled study on relapse and expressed emotion. Arch Gen Psychiatry 43:633–642, 1986

Johnson DAW: Depressions in schizophrenia: some observations on prevalence, etiology, and treatment. Acta Psychiatr Scand 63 (suppl 291):137–144, 1981a

Johnson DAW: Studies of depressive symptoms in schizophrenia. Br J Psychiatry 139:89–101, 1981b

Johnson DAW: The significance of depression in the prediction of relapse in chronic schizophrenia. Br J Psychiatry 152:320–323, 1988

Kessler RC, McGonagle KA, Swartz M, et al: Sex and depression in the National Comorbidity Survey, I: lifetime prevalence, chronicity, and recurrence. J Affect Disord 29:85–96, 1993

Klein DF: Endogenomorphic depression: a conceptual and terminological revision. Arch Gen Psychiatry 31:447–454, 1974

Knights A, Hirsch SR: "Revealed" depression and drug treatment for schizophrenia. Arch Gen Psychiatry 38:806–811, 1981

Koreen AR, Siris SG, Chakos M, et al: Depression in first episode schizophrenia. Am J Psychiatry 150:1643–1648, 1993

Kramer MS, Vogel WH, DiJohnson C, et al: Antidepressants in 'depressed' schizophrenic inpatients: a controlled trial. Arch Gen Psychiatry 46:922–928, 1989

Kuck J, Zisook S, Moranville JT, et al: Negative symptomatology in schizophrenic outpatients. J Nerv Ment Dis 180:510–515, 1992

Kurland AA, Nagaraju A: Viloxazine and the depressed schizophrenic: methodological issues. J Clin Pharmacol 21:37–41, 1981

Lavin MR, Siris SG, Mason SE: What is the clinical importance of cigarette smoking in schizophrenia? Am J Addict 5:189–208, 1996

Leff J, Tress K, Edwards B: The clinical course of depressive symptoms in schizophrenia. Schizophr Res 1:25–30, 1988

Lerner Y, Mintzer Y, Schestatzky M: Lithium combined with haloperidol in schizophrenic patients. Br J Psychiatry 153:359–362, 1988

Levitt JJ, Tsuang MT: The heterogeneity of schizoaffective disorder: implications for treatment. Am J Psychiatry 145:926–936, 1988

Lewine R: Schizophrenia: An amotivational syndrome in men. Can J Psychiatry 30:316–318, 1985

Lindenmayer J-P, Grochowski S, Kay SR: Schizophrenic patients with depression: psychopathological profiles and relationship with negative symptoms. Compr Psychiatry 32:528–533, 1991

Mandel MR, Severe JB, Schooler NR, et al: Development and prediction of postpsychotic depression in neuroleptic-treated schizophrenics. Arch Gen Psychiatry 39:197–203, 1982

Martin RL, Cloninger RC, Guze SB, et al: Frequency and differential diagnosis of depressive syndromes in schizophrenia. J Clin Psychiatry 46 (no 11, sec 2):9–13, 1985

McGlashan TH, Bardenstein KK: Gender differences in affective, schizoaffective, and schizophrenic disorders. Schizophr Bull 16:319–329, 1990

McGlashan TH, Carpenter WT Jr: An investigation of the postpsychotic depressive syndrome. Am J Psychiatry 133:14–19, 1976a

McGlashan TH, Carpenter WJ Jr: Postpsychotic depression in schizophrenia. Arch Gen Psychiatry 33:231–239, 1976b

Miles C: Conditions predisposing to suicide. A review. J Nerv Ment Dis 164:221–246, 1977

Miller JB, Sonnenberg SM: Depression following psychotic episodes: a response to the challenge of change? J Am Acad Psychoanal 1:253–270, 1973

Moller HJ, von Zerssen D: Depressive states occurring during the neuroleptic treatment of schizophrenia. Schizophr Bull 8:109–117, 1982

Moller HJ, von Zerssen D: Handbook of Studies on Schizophrenia. New York, Elsevier, 1986

Norman RMG, Malla AK: Dysphoric mood and symptomatology in schizophrenia. Psychol Med 21:897–903, 1991

Norman RMG, Malla AK: Correlation over time between dysphoric mood and symptomatology in schizophrenia. Compr Psychiatry 35:34–38, 1994

Nuechterlein KH, Dawson MD: A heuristic vulnerability/stress model of schizophrenic episodes. Schizophr Bull 10:300–312, 1984

Perenyi A, Goswami U, Frecska E, et al: L-Deprenyl in treating negative symptoms of schizophrenia. Psychiatry Res 42:189–191, 1992

Plasky P: Antidepressant usage in schizophrenia. Schizophr Bull 17:75–98, 1991

Prasad AJ, Kumar N: Suicidal behavior in hospitalized schizophrenics. Suicide Life Threat Behav 18:265–269, 1988

Prusoff BA, Williams DH, Weissman MM, et al: Treatment of secondary depression in schizophrenia. Arch Gen Psychiatry 36:569–575, 1979

Riecher-Rossler A, Hafner H, Stumbaum M, et al: Can estradiol modulate schizophrenic symptomatology? Schizophr Bull 20:203–214, 1994

Rifkin A, Quitkin F, Klein DF: Akinesia: a poorly recognized drug-induced extrapyramidal behavioral disorder. Arch Gen Psychiatry 32:672–674, 1975

Rifkin A, Quitkin F, Kane JM, et al: Are prophylactic antiparkinson drugs necessary? Arch Gen Psychiatry 35:483–489, 1978

Roth S: The seemingly ubiquitous depression following acute schizophrenic episodes, a neglected area of clinical discussion. Am J Psychiatry 127:51–58, 1970

Roy A: Suicide in chronic schizophrenia. Br J Psychiatry 141:171–177, 1982

Roy A: Do neuroleptics cause depression? Biol Psychiatry 19:777–781, 1984

Roy A: Depression, attempted suicide and suicide in patients with chronic schizophrenia. Psychiatr Clin North Am 9:193–206, 1986

Roy A, Thompson R, Kennedy S: Depression in chronic schizophrenia. Br J Psychiatry 142:465–470, 1983

Sands JR, Harrow M: Depression during the longitudinal course of schizophrenia. Schizophr Bull 25:157–171, 1999

Seeman MV: The role of estrogen in schizophrenia. J Psychiatry Neuroscience 21:123–127, 1996a

Seeman MV: Schizophrenia, gender, and affect. Can J Psychiatry 41:263–264, 1996b

Seeman MV: Psychopathology in women and men: focus on female hormones. Am J Psychiatry 154:1641–1647, 1997

Semrad EV: Long-term therapy of schizophrenia: formulation of the clinical approach, in Psychoneuroses and Schizophrenia. Edited by Usdin GP. Philadelphia, PA, JB Lippincott, 1966, pp 155-173

Shear K, Frances A, Weiden P: Suicide associated with akathisia and depot fluphenazine treatment. J Clin Psychopharmacol 3:235–236, 1983

Shtasel DL, Gur RE, Gallacher F, et al: Gender differences in the clinical expression of schizophrenia. Schizophr Res 7:225–231, 1992

Silver H, Nassar A: Fluvoxamine improves negative symptoms in treated chronic schizophrenia: an add-on double-blind, placebo-controlled study. Biol Psychiatry 31:698–704, 1992

Singh AN, Saxena B, Nelson HL: A controlled clinical study of trazodone in chronic schizophrenic patients with pronounced depressive symptomatology. Current Therapeutics Research 23:485–501, 1978

Siris SG: Akathisia and "acting-out." J Clin Psychiatry 46:395–397, 1985

Siris SG: Implications of normal brain development for the pathogenesis of schizophrenia (letter). Arch Gen Psychiatry 45:1055, 1988

Siris SG: Diagnosis of secondary depression in schizophrenia: implications for DSM-IV. Schizophr Bull 17.75–98, 1991

Siris SG: Depression and schizophrenia, in Schizophrenia. Edited by Hirsch SR, Weinberger DR. Cambridge, MA, Blackwell Science, 1995, pp 128–145

Siris SG: The treatment of schizoaffective disorder, in Current Psychiatric Therapy II. Edited by Dunner DL. Philadelphia, PA, WB Saunders, 1996, pp 196–201

Siris SG: Depression in schizophrenia: perspective in the era of "atypical" antipsychotic agents. Am J Psychiatry 157:1379–1389, 2000

Siris SG, Lavin MR: Schizoaffective disorder, schizophreniform disorder and acute psychotic disorder (including brief reactive psychosis), in Comprehensive Textbook of Psychiatry/VI, 6th Edition. Edited by Kaplan HI, Sadock BJ. Philadelphia, PA, Williams & Wilkins, 1995, pp 1019–1031

Siris SG, Morgan V, Fagerstrom R, et al: Adjunctive imipramine in the treatment of post-psychotic depression: a controlled trial. Arch Gen Psychiatry 44:533–539, 1987

Siris SG, Adan F, Cohen M, et al: Post-psychotic depression and negative symptoms: an investigation of syndromal overlap. Am J Psychiatry 145:1532–1537, 1988a

Siris SG, Strahan A, Mandeli J, et al: Fluphenazine decanoate dose and severity of depression in patients with post-psychotic depression. Schizophr Res 1:31–35, 1988b

Siris SG, Bermanzohn PC, Mason SE, et al: Maintenance imipramine therapy for secondary depression in schizophrenia: a controlled trial. Arch Gen Psychiatry 51:109–115, 1994

Spina E, DeDomenico P, Ruello C, et al: Adjunctive fluoxetine in the treatment of negative symptoms in chronic schizophrenic patients. Int Clin Psychopharmacol 9:281–285, 1994

Spitzer RL, Endicott J, Robins E: Research Diagnostic Criteria: rationale and reliability. Arch Gen Psychiatry 35:773–782, 1978

Stephens JH, Richard P, McHugh PR: Suicide in patients hospitalized for schizophrenia: 1913–1940. J Nerv Ment Dis 187:10–14, 1999

Strian F, Heger R, Klicpera C: The time structure of depressive mood in schizophrenic patients. Acta Psychiatr Scand 65:66–73, 1982

Szymanski HV, Simon J, Gutterman N: Recovery from schizophrenic psychosis. Am J Psychiatry 140:335–338, 1983

Tapp A, Tandon R, Douglass A, et al: Depression in severe chronic schizophrenia. Biol Psychiatry 35:667, 1994

Taylor MA: Are schizophrenia and affective disorder related? A selective literature review. Am J Psychiatry 149:22–32, 1992

Tollefson GD, Andersen SW, Tran PV: The course of depressive symptoms in predicting relapse in schizophrenia: a double-blind, randomized comparison of olanzapine and risperidone. Biol Psychiatry 46:365–373, 1999

Van Putten T: The many faces of akathisia. Compr Psychiatry 16:43–47, 1975

Van Putten T, May PRA: 'Akinetic depression' in schizophrenia. Arch Gen Psychiatry 35:1101–1107, 1978

Waehrens J, Gerlach J: Antidepressant drugs in anergic schizophrenia: a double-blind cross-over study with maprotiline and placebo. Acta Psychiatr Scand 61:438–444, 1980

Weinberger DR: Implications of normal brain development for the pathogenesis of schizophrenia. Arch Gen Psychiatry 44:660–669, 1987

Winokur G: Family history studies, VIII: secondary depression is alive and well, and . . . Diseases of the Nervous System 33:94–99, 1972

Wise RA: Neuroleptics and operant behaviour: the anhedonia hypothesis. Behav Brain Sci 5:39–87, 1982

Wistedt B, Palmstierna T: Depressive symptoms in chronic schizophrenic patients after withdrawal of long-acting neuroleptics. J Clin Psychiatry 44:369–371, 1983

World Health Organization: International Classification of Diseases (ICD-10): Clinical Descriptions and Diagnostic Guidelines (draft of field trials). Geneva, World Health Organization, 1988

Zubin J, Spring B: Vulnerability: a new view of schizophrenia. J Abnorm Psychol 86:103–126, 1977

CHAPTER 3

Obsessive-Compulsive Symptoms in Patients With Schizophrenia

Michael Y. Hwang, M.D.
Paul C. Bermanzohn, M.D.
Lewis A. Opler, M.D., Ph.D.

*T*he relationship between obsessive-compulsive disorder (OCD) and schizophrenia has intrigued clinicians for over a century. Because obsessive-compulsive (OC) phenomena may resemble and become intertwined with psychotic phenomena, patients exhibiting this clinical overlap have been difficult to recognize and to treat. Not surprisingly, there have been few studies to establish optimal therapies for this complex group of patients. Findings from more definitive clinical and biological studies are still awaited. In this chapter, we review what is currently known about the diagnosis and treatment of schizophrenia with OC symptoms, a condition we refer to as "OC-schizophrenia."

Many early clinicians thought that OC phenomena were a part of schizophrenia and proposed various explanations for this (Bleuler 1911/1950; Bumke 1944; A. Freud 1966; S. Freud 1908/1957; Westphal 1878). Several clinical reports (Rosen 1957; Stengel 1945) found that the patients

Preparation of this chapter was supported in part by a postdoctoral training grant through National Research Service Award of the National Institute of Mental Health (Dr. Hwang).

with OC-schizophrenia had a comparatively benign clinical course and better outcome. This led to the suggestion that OC symptoms are protective and that persons undergoing a schizophrenic break develop OC symptoms as a defense against psychotic disorganization. More recent studies, however, seem to contradict these earlier beliefs that OC symptoms are protective. Rather, these studies found that schizophrenia patients with OC symptoms have poorer global functioning and outcome (Berman et al. 1995; Fenton and McGlashan 1986), as well as greater neuropsychiatric impairments (Hwang and Hollander 1992; Hwang et al. 2000; Samuels et al. 1993) than schizophrenia patients without OC symptoms, suggesting that significant OC symptoms in patients with schizophrenia may predict a worse long-term outcome. Furthermore, the estimates of the prevalence of OC symptoms in schizophrenia have increased in recent years.

Given that OC-schizophrenia appears to be both common and disabling, the lack of systematic studies on this condition comes as a surprise. The dearth of treatment studies has been due, at least in part, to difficulty recognizing such cases, as well as lack of effective treatment for OC-schizophrenia. Clinical studies and treatment guidelines for OC-schizophrenia are needed to guide clinicians in the management of this condition.

In this chapter, we review the existing literature and propose tentative treatment guidelines to assist the practitioner. These guidelines are subject to revision as more definitive studies become available.

Recognition of Obsessive-Compulsive Symptoms in Patients With Schizophrenia

Phenomenology

Obsessions are generally thought to be distinct and separable from psychotic phenomena in schizophrenia, but the distinction is often difficult to make clinically. Both obsessions and delusions rest on false, absurd, or excessive ideas, and they are supposed to be distinguishable on the basis of insight. Clinical wisdom on this point is simple and clear. Obsessions are ego dystonic, and delusions are ego syntonic. Patients with obsessions recognize the obsessions as coming from their own mind and resist these preoccupations as pathological intrusions. Delusions, on the other hand, are believed and embraced by the patient. Thus, the distinction between obsessions and delusions is clearly made on the basis of the preservation of insight and ability to resist the intrusive thoughts and/or behaviors.

Psychotic Obsessions

Unfortunately, such simple and sharp distinctions may break down in actual clinical practice. Earlier clinicians coined various terms to describe patients with poor insight who show little or no resistance to, or insight into, the absurdity of the OC symptoms as a "psychotic or malignant form of OCD." The problem has been most extensively studied in OCD (Solyom et al. 1985). Evidence indicates that the insight and resistance in OCD is neither universal nor constant and that patients with obsessions often lose insight into the pathological nature of their preoccupations. Foa and Kozak (1995) found that "a large majority" of patients with OCD experience some loss of insight at least some of the time. Obsessional patients may exhibit a spectrum of insight into their obsessions, varying from fully intact insight to a complete loss of insight. Those with a complete loss of insight are said to have "psychotic OCD" (Solyom et al. 1985; see also Insel and Akiskal 1986).

Further complicating this clinical distinction are the reports of obsessions with a psychotic theme in patients with chronic schizophrenia. These obsessive delusions appear to be hybrid phenomena, obsessive in form and psychotic in content; obsessive delusions may not be cross sectionally distinguishable from schizophrenic phenomena (Bermanzohn et al. 1997).

Recovering Delusions

Delusional patients also may exhibit great variability of insight. Kendler et al. (1983) pointed out that "often patients (with delusions) do not have absolute conviction." Patients may report they no longer have "those crazy thoughts" or that they still have them but no longer believe them. Spitzer (1985) called such phenomena "recovering delusions" and proposed stages in the recovery process. As the patient recovers, there is a progression of stages from the delusion's being maintained with full conviction to the delusion's having no effect on the patient's everyday life. As these patients recover more fully, there may be a reduction of certainty about the delusion until, finally, the delusion is only remembered but with no claim as to its truth. This description of variations in insight with the delusion has not been systematically studied (Ghaemi and Pope 1994).

With such variability in insight in both obsessions and delusions, insight does not appear to provide a reliable basis on which to distinguish between obsessions and delusions. Obsessions and delusions on occasion may overlap (Bermanzohn et al. 1997), making it difficult to recognize OC symptoms in patients with schizophrenia. Obsessions may become delusional in the manner just described and so may be taken for purely schizophrenic delusions. This is likely to affect attempts to determine the frequency with which OC symptoms occur in schizophrenia.

Epidemiology

The rates for OC symptoms occurring in patients with schizophrenia have varied widely. Reported rates have ranged from 1.1% (Jahrreiss 1926) to 59.2% (Bland et al. 1987). These estimates have varied so widely because, in addition to the difficulty in distinguishing obsessive from delusional phenomena, different patient samples and definitions of OCD and of schizophrenia were used, and studies differed as to whether they looked for only OC symptoms or full OCD and whether they reported lifetime or point prevalence (see Table 3–1).

In any case, there has been an increase in the rate at which OC phenomena are reported among patients with schizophrenia. This parallels the increasing frequency of the diagnosis of OCD in the general population (Karno et al. 1988; Regier et al. 1988). This increase in the frequency of the diagnosis of OCD probably stems from a greater willingness by clinicians to make the diagnosis as effective treatments for OCD have become available (Stoll et al. 1992). It also appears that OC symptoms in patients with schizophrenia occur more commonly than OCD in the general population, in which the prevalence of the disorder is approximately 2.5% (see Chapter 1, Table 1–1). Yet, although there have been remarkable advances in the neurobiology and pharmacological treatment of OCD, surprisingly few systematic studies have attempted to apply these new advances in OC-schizophrenia.

OC-Schizophrenia as a Subtype in Schizophrenic Spectrum Disorder

Zohar (1997) proposed a "schizo-obsessive" subtype of schizophrenia, and others have supported a similar view based on pharmacological response data (Table 3–2) and on epidemiological data (Table 3–1). In an earlier study, Hwang et al. (1992, 2000) investigated the clinical and neuropsychological profiles of patients with OC-schizophrenia, comparing them with the profiles of a group of patients with schizophrenia but no OC symptoms matched for age, sex, and duration of illness. The authors found that the OC-schizophrenia group demonstrated significantly greater neuropsychological (prefrontal executive functioning) and psychopathological (negative symptoms) impairments. This finding supported the results of earlier reports that indicated positive correlations between greater prefrontal dysfunction/higher negative symptoms and poor clinical course in chronic schizophrenia (Butler et al. 1992; Opler et al. 1991).

On the other hand, Berman et al. (1997) found that the cognitive deficits in OC-schizophrenia patients are similar to those in patients with

Table 3–1. Prevalence estimates for obsessive-compulsive disorder (OCD) and obsessive-compulsive (OC) symptoms in patients with schizophrenia

Report	Methods and criteria	Sample	Results
Jahrreiss 1926	Chart review with strict criteria for OCD but not for schizophrenia	1,000 charts of hospitalized and clinic patients	11 patients met criteria for OCD; prevalence rate of 11%
Rosen 1957	Chart review without specified criteria for either OCD or schizophrenia	Studied 848 charts of hospitalized inpatients	30 patients (3.5%) had OCD "at some time"
Fenton and McGlashan 1986	Chart review with follow-up an average of 15 years later DSM-III-R criteria[a] for schizophrenia with behavioral criteria for OC symptoms	Followed up 163 inpatients	21 patients (12.9%) met two of eight behavioral criteria for OC symptoms
Bland et al. 1987	Random community survey using DIS and DSM-III[b] criteria for both schizophrenia and OCD	Interviewed 2,144 community residents and found 20 with DIS/DSM-III schizophrenia	11 patients met DIS/DSM-III criteria for OCD (statistically corrected to 59.2%)
Berman et al. 1995	Structured interviews of patient therapists at CMHC; chart diagnoses for schizophrenia and criteria of Fenton and McGlashan (1986) for OC symptoms	Interviewed therapists of 108 CMHC patients with chronic schizophrenia	27 patients exhibited OC symptoms during study (26.5% point prevalence); 33 patients had OC symptoms at any time (30.6% lifetime prevalence)

Table 3–1. Prevalence estimates for obsessive-compulsive disorder (OCD) and obsessive-compulsive (OC) symptoms in patients with schizophrenia (*continued*)

Report	Methods and criteria	Sample	Results
D. S. Rae, unpublished data, 1996	Reanalysis of ECA survey: random community survey of five U.S. communities using DIS and DSM-III criteria for both schizophrenia and OCD		Prevalence of OCD: 23.7%
Bermanzohn et al. 2000	Lifetime prevalence study, using SCID-IV, of schizophrenia and schizoaffective patients with OC symptoms and OCD	Interviewed 37 chronic schizophrenia patients in comprehensive day program	Lifetime prevalences: OC symptoms: 43.2% (*n* = 16) OCD: 29.7% (*n* = 11)
Porto et al. 1997	Lifetime prevalence study, using DSM-IV SCID, of schizophrenia and schizoaffective patients with OC symptoms and OCD	Interviewed 50 chronic schizophrenia patients in comprehensive day program	Lifetime prevalences: "Clinically significant" OC symptoms: 43.2% (*n* = 30) Full OCD: 29.7%
Eisen et al. 1997	Lifetime prevalence study, using DSM-III-R SCID, of schizophrenia and schizoaffective patients	Interviewed 77 clinic outpatients with schizophrenia or schizoaffective disorder	Lifetime prevalence: OCD: 7.8% (*n* = 6)

Table 3–1. Prevalence estimates for obsessive-compulsive disorder (OCD) and obsessive-compulsive (OC) symptoms in patients with schizophrenia (*continued*)

Report	Methods and criteria	Sample	Results
Meghani et al. 1998	All new admissions to an outpatient psychiatry service in a large midwestern teaching hospital over 5 years (*N* = 1,458) were administered structured diagnostic instrument and self-report measures	31.7% (*n* = 61) of all schizophrenia patients (*N* = 192) met criteria for OCD.	Patients with OCD-schizophrenia had "less efficient psychosocial functioning" and "lower self-satisfaction"; no treatment differences between the two groups noted except that OCD-schizophrenia patients were more likely to say that the medications they received "made no difference"

Note. CMHC = community mental health center; DIS = Diagnostic Interview Schedule; ECA = Epidemiologic Catchment Area; SCID = Structured Clinical Interview for DSM.
[a] American Psychiatric Association 1987.
[b] American Psychiatric Association 1980.
[c] Bland et al. used a standard statistical correction for household size.

OCD alone (impaired visual-spatial skills, delayed visual memory, and impaired capacity to shift cognitive sets) and that these patients respond to treatment with anti-obsessional agents. From these data, they concluded that OC symptoms in schizophrenia are more similar to OCD than to schizophrenia and that they are distinct from schizophrenic symptoms. On the basis of their findings of more floridly psychotic symptoms, greater neuropsychological impairment, and longer hospitalizations among patients with OC-schizophrenia, some clinicians have argued that these patients may constitute a distinct schizophrenia subgroup (Hwang and Opler 1994; Samuels et al. 1993).

Although we support the use of subtyping strategies, the use of terms like "schizo-obsessive" should be avoided, because such a label, though descriptive, would introduce more confusion than clarification into our present attempts to conceptualize the co-occurrence of OC phenomena with schizophrenia.

Clinical Features

Differential Diagnosis

From a literature review and clinical experience, Hwang and Opler (1994) identified three groups of schizophrenia patients with delusional OC phenomena. The first group comprises patients with long-standing OC symptoms prior to the onset of psychosis. These patients begin with DSM-IV-diagnosable OCD and subsequently develop delusional obsessions in the course of chronic and treatment-refractory illness. They may exhibit varying degrees of insight into and resistance to their diverse OC symptoms. Patients in this category previously have met the criteria for OCD and currently may meet the criteria for schizophrenia. These patients also have been traditionally referred to as having "psychotic or malignant" OCD.

The second group consists of patients with OC symptoms whose onset is concurrent with or follows the onset of DSM-diagnosable schizophrenia. These patients have an unequivocal diagnosis of schizophrenia and may have little or no insight into their OC symptoms. They often display a worse clinical course and poorer treatment outcome than do schizophrenia patients without OC symptoms.

The third group constitutes patients with well-established schizophrenia who present with transient and varied OC symptoms during the course of their schizophrenic illness. These patients usually show poor or no insight into their OC symptoms.

Prognosis

Earlier it was thought that OC symptoms served as a defense against psychotic decompensation. On the basis of case reports (Stengel 1945) and uncontrolled retrospective chart reviews (Rosen 1957), it was suggested that OC symptoms attenuate the schizophrenic illness and make for a less virulent course. More recent systematic studies, however, have found the contrary. Fenton and McGlashan (1986), following up 163 schizophrenia patients an average of 15 years after an index admission as part of the Chestnut Lodge Follow-Up Study, found that OC symptoms in 21 patients were associated with a global decline in function relative to the function of 142 patients without OC symptoms. Berman et al. (1995) questioned the therapists of 108 chronic schizophrenia patients about the presence of OC symptoms and the patients' functioning and found that OC patients were judged to have a lower capacity for age-appropriate function, confirming Fenton and McGlashan's (1986) findings. Samuels et al. (1993) also found that 66 schizophrenia patients with OC symptoms had "more florid presentation of symptom[s] with earlier age of onset of psychosis and a greater number of hospitalizations" than the 283 patients without OC symptoms.

Treatment of OC Symptoms in Patients With Schizophrenia

Until recently, there has been only limited recognition of OC symptoms in patients with schizophrenia, and, perhaps, for this reason limited pharmacological treatment studies have been done. Clomipramine and selective serotonin reuptake inhibitors (SSRIs) found to be effective in the treatment of OCD and related disorders (Greist et al. 1995; Hollander 1993) also have been used as an adjunctive treatment in patients with OC-schizophrenia in recent years.

Adjunctive Anti-OC Medications

Early anecdotal case reports and open treatment studies with clomipramine suggested mostly positive, but some negative, outcome findings for the use of adjunctive anti-OC medications in the treatment of patients with OC-schizophrenia. Subsequently, Hwang and colleagues (Hwang and Opler 1994; Hwang et al. 1993, 1995), in a series of open treatment studies, found a significant clinical and neuropsychological improvement when an SSRI was added to a stable antipsychotic regimen in patients with previously refractory OC-schizophrenia. Furthermore, they noted that the OC symptoms may respond independently from psychotic symptoms and that the optimal individual SSRI dose varied from patient to patient.

Although there have been a number of anecdotal case reports on the use of adjunctive anti-OC medication in the treatment of OC-schizophrenia, we summarize here five treatment studies. Although the studies include somewhat different patient populations with varying clinical information and study criteria, we draw some tentative conclusions (see Table 3–2).

Most of the studies of treating OC symptoms in schizophrenia patients reported thus far (and several of these are actually multiple case reports rather than systematic studies) have used clomipramine and have yielded generally positive findings about its clinical effects. (For a review of case reports in treatment of OC symptoms in schizophrenia, see Sasson et al. 1997.)

1. In an early study of clomipramine in the treatment of OCD, Yaryura-Tobias et al. (1976) openly treated 10 outpatients with schizophrenia and OC symptoms. Even though neuroleptics could be used ad libitum, 4 of the 10 patients experienced an exacerbation of psychosis. The 6 remaining patients who were able to tolerate the 8-week trial experienced a reduction in anxiety, particularly anxiety associated with rituals. No other changes were noted. On the basis of the psychotic exacerbation found in 4 patients, the authors concluded that clomipramine should be given to patients with psychosis "with caution, concomitant with neuroleptic medication, and only where the severity of OC symptoms makes the treatment imperative"(p. 545) However, since there was no control group, it is impossible to say if relapses to psychosis occurred at a rate greater than a spontaneous rate.

2. Pulman et al. (1984) reported the results of an "informal," open trial in which clomipramine was given to six hospitalized patients with chronic schizophrenia, three of whom showed no insight into their OC symptoms. Four patients showed an improvement in their OC symptoms, and another experienced an exacerbation of psychosis. Unfortunately, the doses and duration of treatment were not specified and the conditions were uncontrolled, making this report difficult to interpret.

3. Stroebel et al. (1984), in an open trial, gave clomipramine to 17 schizophrenia outpatients with OC symptoms as part of a larger report on their experience using clomipramine in the treatment of OCD. Other medications were not held constant, and the duration of treatment was not specified but was described only as lasting "up to 757 days." Seven patients (41%) showed improvement in their OC symptoms,

Table 3–2. Treatment trials of clomipramine for obsessive-compulsive symptoms in patients with schizophrenia

Report	Sample	Design	Duration	Ratings	Psychosis	OC symptoms	Comments
Berman et al. 1995	6 stable outpatients	Double-blind, crossover	13 weeks	PANSS, Y-BOCS, CGI	Improved	Improved	
Pulman et al. 1984[a]	8 chronically hospitalized patients; OC symptoms not part of a "classical OCD neurosis"; three with no resistance to OC symptoms	"Informal" open	No set time	None	Exacerbated in 4 patients	Improved in 4 patients	Case reports; not a controlled trial
Stroebel et al. 1984[a]	17	Open; other medications not held constant (>1 on no neuroleptics)	Up to 757 days		Worse in 4 patients (>1 taking no neuroleptics; 3 taking "low" doses of neuroleptic)	Improved in 7 patients	Poorly designed

Table 3–2. Treatment trials of clomipramine for obsessive-compulsive symptoms in patients with schizophrenia *(continued)*

Report	Sample	Design	Duration	Ratings	Psychosis	OC symptoms	Comments
Yaryura-Tobias et al. 1976[a]	10	Open; neuroleptics given ad libitum	8 weeks	CGI, Ham-D, BPRS, OCI	4 dropped because of increased psychotic symptoms	Reduced anxiety with rituals; no other significant changes	
Zohar et al. 1993	3 with schizophrenia; 2 with schizoaffective disorder	Open ABA	>6 weeks	BPRS, Y-BOCS	Diminished in 4 patients; increased in 1 patient	Decreased in 5 patients	Case reports

Note. BPRS = Brief Psychiatric Rating Scale; CGI = Clinical Global Improvement; Ham-D = Hamilton Rating Scale for Depression; OC = obsessive-compulsive; OCD = obsessive-compulsive disorder; OCI = Obsessive-Compulsive Symptom Inventory; PANSS = Positive and Negative Syndrome Scale; Y-BOCS = Yale-Brown Obsessive Compulsive Scale.
[a]Schizophrenia patients with OCD were part of a larger study of clomipramine for OCD.

and although "at least 1" patient was not receiving neuroleptic medication at some time during the trial, 4 experienced a worsening of psychosis. It is not clear how many of these patients were not receiving neuroleptics. The lack of systematization in the reporting of the data, as well as the lack of symptom scales to rate symptom severity, limits the utility of this report.

4. Zohar et al. (1993) reported the results of an open trial in which clomipramine was administered to five patients, three with a diagnosis of schizophrenia and two diagnosed with schizoaffective disorder for a period lasting greater than 6 weeks. The clomipramine was stopped and then started again, and the patients were systematically rated during the course of these changes. In all five patients, the OC symptoms diminished. Four of the five patients also experienced a reduction in psychotic symptoms, whereas one patient had an exacerbation of psychotic symptoms.

5. The best-controlled study reported thus far of the treatment of OC symptoms in patients with schizophrenia is a pilot study by Berman et al. (1995), in which clomipramine was administered to six stable outpatients in a double-blind, crossover trial. Under double-blind conditions, patients were first given either placebo or active clomipramine and then switched to the other agent. This crossover design allowed patients to act as their own controls. Patients who were taking low-potency neuroleptics such as chlorpromazine or thioridazine were excluded because it was feared that the anticholinergic effects of the clomipramine might be additive with those of the neuroleptic. Patients improved significantly more when receiving clomipramine than when receiving placebo. All six patients also showed a reduction in psychotic symptoms.

We would like to underscore that the positive treatment response with adjunctive anti-OC medication has not been universally observed. For example, Lindenmayer et al. (1990) and Bark and Lindenmayer (1992) reported that treatment with adjunctive SSRI failed to improve OC symptoms and exacerbated psychotic symptoms, although objective measures of OC symptom severity were not used in their assessments.

Effect of New Antipsychotics on OC-Schizophrenia: An Ongoing Debate

There has been debate over whether OC symptoms are affected in some way by the new generation of antipsychotic medications. There have been a number of case reports of patients receiving new-generation antipsychotics, especially clozapine and risperidone, either developing new or experiencing a worsening of old OC symptoms (Baker et al. 1997). Such clinical developments have been explained by the central serotonergic receptor blocking effects of the newer antipsychotics (decreased central serotonergic activity has been implicated in the etiology of OCD). Patel and Tandon (1993) treated two schizophrenia patients who developed clozapine-induced OC symptoms with adjunctive fluoxetine and found a reduction in the OC symptoms with no increase in psychotic symptoms. Similarly, Allen and Tejera (1994) successfully treated one schizophrenia patient who developed OC symptoms while being treated with clozapine; the patient experienced a reduction in OC symptoms without any exacerbation of psychosis or significant side effects.

On the other hand, Ghaemi et al. (1995) reviewed the charts of 142 patients who had begun receiving clozapine at McLean Hospital and failed to find evidence of an increase in or onset of new OC symptoms among these patients. Furthermore, Bermanzohn et al. (1997) described two patients whose OC-schizophrenia improved after administration of clozapine. Similarly, McDougle et al. (1995) reported success with the adjunctive risperidone treatment in patients with previously treatment-refractory OCD.

These conflicting reports have created some uncertainty about the use of atypical antipsychotics in schizophrenia patients with OC symptoms. Prospective controlled studies are needed to determine the role of the atypical antipsychotics in OC-schizophrenia.

Provisional Recommendations for Treatment of OC-Schizophrenia

Given the current state of knowledge regarding the pharmacotherapy of OC symptoms in patients with schizophrenia, with all the strengths and limitations of the few studies and clinical reports available at present, several tentative recommendations can be made.

- Anti-obsessional agents should be selected on the basis of their pharmacokinetics and their profile of side effects and how these medication effects might be expected to interact with the primary antipsychotic pharmacotherapy (Siris 1993). Of particular concern is the ability of many of these compounds to induce or exacerbate agitation or akathisia. Additionally, anticholinergic effects are common to both clomipramine and some of the newer-generation antipsychotics, in particular clozapine. Both clozapine and clomipramine block α-adrenergic receptors, with the concomitant side effects (e.g., sedation and hypotension), and lower the seizure threshold. Finally, SSRIs appear to increase the blood levels of typical neuroleptics by as much as 25%–30% while causing an even greater increase in clozapine (Ciraulo and Shader 1990; Goff et al. 1991). Therefore, clinicians must carefully monitor patients for potential adverse effects due to both pharmacodynamic and pharmacokinetic drug-drug interactions.

- Patients receiving clozapine as their maintenance neuroleptic should be assessed to determine, if possible, whether their OC symptoms preceded the start of clozapine therapy. If the OC symptoms appear to have started or worsened with the institution of clozapine treatment, the clinician might consider switching to another atypical antipsychotic after carefully weighing the benefits derived from clozapine against the morbidity caused by an increase in OC symptoms. If clozapine is to be continued, SSRIs might be the anti-obsessional treatment of choice, given the problems associated with combining clozapine with clomipramine.
- Finally, for optimum outcome, pharmacotherapy should be combined with the cognitive and behavioral psychotherapy in treating OC-schizophrenia.

Clinical Cases

Case 1

A 45-year-old, single male presented with a 27-year history of chronic undifferentiated schizophrenia, including 16 years of institutionalization. On his last hospital admission, 4 years previously, he was agitated and psychotic, as well as engaged in a number of bizarre, stereotyped behaviors (e.g., repeatedly washing face and hands; touching door frames in a ritualistic manner before walking through them). His symptoms remained unchanged or worse during the next year, despite trials of various neuroleptics, both alone and in combination with lithium, carbamazepine, propranolol, and lorazepam. A neurology consult, including electroencephalogram (EEG), brain computed tomography (CT) scan, and skull series, was unremarkable. Treatment with chlorpromazine 1,000 mg bid resulted in partial improvement in his psychosis, and the patient benefited from its sedating effects. The bizarre rituals persisted, however, and therefore a clinical trial of fluoxetine was started. After 2 weeks of treatment at 40 mg/day, the patient's rituals became less frequent and intense. His self-care skills improved, and he became more responsive to ward routines and to staff attempts to engage him in therapeutic activities. After a year of treatment, fluoxetine was reduced to 20 mg/day, resulting in a prompt increase in the frequency and intensity of his rituals. Subsequent increase to 60 mg/day of fluoxetine for 6 weeks brought about significant symptom improvement. The patient has remained markedly improved during the past 2 years with chlorpromazine and fluoxetine treatment.

Case 2

A 36-year-old single man with a diagnosis of chronic undifferentiated schizophrenia had his first psychotic decompensation at age 18, with bizarre and persecutory delusions, hallucinations, and both impulsive and compulsive behaviors in response to intrusive thoughts. Subsequently, he had multiple hospitalizations and was treated with a variety of neuroleptics without significant clinical improvement. In addition, he began to exhibit repetitive behaviors such as touching objects in a ritualistic manner, dressing and undressing, and repeatedly smearing body parts with soap and water. These ritualistic behaviors began 3–4 years after the onset of his schizophrenic symptoms.

During his current hospitalization, he was treated with a wide range of neuroleptics as well as a variety of adjunctive medications. Adequate trials of fluoxetine and clomipramine in conjunction with neuroleptics brought about increased levels of anxiety, restlessness, and agitation. Because of the treatment-refractory clinical course, the patient was also treated with clozapine and risperidone. Institution of clozapine treatment was quickly followed by increased agitation and exacerbation of impulsive and compulsive behaviors, causing severe management difficulties. Discontinuation from clozapine resulted in less impulsive and ritualistic behaviors. Risperidone treatment resulted in no substantial symptom improvements, and the patient was unable to tolerate its side effects. Repeated medical and neurological studies, including brain CT scan, were unremarkable.

Case 3

A 35-year-old single man had been diagnosed at age 12 with undifferentiated schizophrenia consisting of hallucinations and paranoid delusions. Since then, he had several relapses that responded well to neuroleptic treatment. His last hospitalization was precipitated by acute paranoid delusions, auditory/visual hallucinations, and catatonic behavior. However, unlike prior relapses, he responded poorly to several neuroleptics and adjunctive medications, remaining markedly psychotic and dysfunctional. Additionally, he began to exhibit bizarre, compulsive rituals that included repetitive touching of objects, opening and closing of doors, drinking water, and forcefully rubbing and injuring his own eyes. His neurological examination, including brain CT scan, was negative. Clomipramine (25 mg/day) was subsequently added to ongoing fluphenazine decanoate (50 mg/2 weeks) and lithium carbonate (1,200 mg/day) treatment and gradually increased to 50 mg/day over 2 weeks. After 4 weeks of treatment with clomipramine at 50 mg/day, his rituals became much less frequent and less intense, allowing improved socialization and participation in various therapeutic activities. However, when the clomipramine was further increased to 150 mg/day, he became restless, hyperactive, impulsive, and agitated. Subsequent dose reduction to 50 mg/day once again resulted in a substantial symptom relief and functional improvements. Over the subsequent 2 years he continued to improve and was discharged.

Discussion

Few systematic studies have carefully studied the implications of OC features in patients with schizophrenia. This has been due, in part, to the earlier diagnostic practices. Specifically, OC symptoms were traditionally regarded as nonpsychotic, anxiety-related phenomena, and earlier diagnostic systems even precluded making a diagnosis of OCD in the presence of schizophrenia. Additionally, until recently, the lack of effective treatment for OC symptoms made their assessment of little immediate clinical relevance.

Recent progress in our understanding of the neurobiology of both schizophrenia and OCD, as well as new advances in their treatment, along with the development of diagnostic criteria (DSM-IV [American Psychiatric Association 1994]) that permit additional Axis I diagnoses to be made in the presence of schizophrenia, has led to increased interest in and attention to the OC phenomena in schizophrenia. Contrary to earlier beliefs that OC-schizophrenia is rare and has a relatively benign clinical course, recent studies suggest significant prevalence and, compared with schizophrenia in the absence of OC features, more ominous clinical course and outcome.

Furthermore, as illustrated in the clinical cases presented in this chapter, patients with OC-schizophrenia have varied clinical presentations as well as responses to anti-OC pharmacotherapy. The patient described in case 1, who has chronic, treatment-refractory, severe OC-schizophrenia, responded well to the adjunctive anti-OC medication. He had a marked clinical and functional improvement associated with OC symptom reduction on a high dose of fluoxetine. The patient in case 2, in contrast, showed a poor response to adjunctive fluoxetine. He also had an adverse response to both clozapine and risperidone, with increased anxiety and impulsive, compulsive behaviors. The patient in case 3 exhibited a marked reduction in OC symptoms and functional improvement on low-dose (50 mg) clomipramine treatment. He became acutely agitated, exhibiting markedly increased impulsive and ritualistic behaviors on a higher dose (150 mg) of clomipramine; his symptoms once again improved on returning to a low-dose (50 mg/day) regimen. Interestingly, in this patient, OC symptom reduction correlated well with clinical and neuropsychological improvement but was independent of changes in positive psychotic symptoms; this suggests that OC features and positive symptoms may reflect different dimensions of psychopathology in schizophrenia. This differential treatment response is consistent with our earlier speculation that OC symptoms in schizophrenia arise from a coexisting neurobiological process that is independent of those processes that lead to psychotic symptoms in schizophrenia (Hwang et al. 1995).

Although further controlled studies are needed to establish the therapeutic efficacy of the adjunctive anti-OC pharmacotherapy, preliminary findings suggest that some patients with OC-schizophrenia benefit from this treatment. In combining antipsychotic and anti-OC medications, however, clinicians must be aware of both pharmacokinetic and pharmacodynamic drug-drug interactions. All SSRIs competitively inhibit microsomal P450 isoenzymes in the human liver. In both preclinical and clinical studies, fluoxetine (and its active metabolite, norfluoxetine), as well as other SSRIs, substantially increased tricyclic antidepressant and antipsychotic blood levels (Ciraulo and Shader 1990; Goff et al. 1991). Additionally, SSRIs can cause or exacerbate akathisia and other extrapyramidal symptoms, worsening motor side effects if combined with standard neuroleptics. Hence, the use of an SSRI as an adjunctive therapy for patients with OC-schizophrenia must be based on careful medical and pharmacological considerations.

Our review of neurobiological studies in schizophrenia and OCD has failed to establish evidence for a single shared pathogenic mechanism. Whereas OCD appears to involve serotonergic dysregulation and disruptions in basal ganglia that modulate activities between the orbitofrontal cortex and limbic striatal circuits, schizophrenia entails far more pervasive and varied central nervous system (CNS) involvement, including the frontal, parietal, temporal, cingulate, and limbic regions. Recent advances in the understanding of CNS dopamine-serotonin interactions and the advent of the effective combined serotonin and dopamine antagonists in the pharmacotherapy of schizophrenia suggest multisystem involvement in that disorder. Further, the coexistence of OCD and schizophrenia symptoms, and the specific response of OC symptoms to SSRI treatment, suggest a distinct neurobiological basis for the OC symptoms in OC-schizophrenia. Given that, at present, it is not clear whether this subgroup of patients are best conceptualized as having a distinct schizophrenia subtype, as having schizophrenia with a prominent OC dimension, or as having comorbid OCD and schizophrenia, all three of these models should be considered in evaluating and treating patients with OC-schizophrenia.

Summary

Although OC phenomena have long been recognized in patients with schizophrenia, few systematic studies have examined their clinical and neurobiological significance. Recent epidemiological and clinical studies indicate, first, a significant prevalence of OC-schizophrenia and, second, greater neuropsychological impairments and poorer clinical course in patients with this condition. Recent treatment studies have shown that combining anti-OC medications with either standard neuroleptics or atypical antipsychotics, while monitoring blood levels and side effects in light of complex drug-drug interactions, may lead to improved outcomes and better quality of life for this difficult-to-treat group of schizophrenia patients.

It should be noted that there have been no specific studies to examine the epidemiological or clinical profiles of female patients with OC-schizophrenia. However, increasing evidence suggests significant gender differences in schizophrenic illness. Hence, we recommend that clinicians carefully consider various factors, such as gestational and endocrinological status, in the management of OC-schizophrenia in female patients (see Chapter 6, this volume).

Our conclusions are necessarily tentative. In our review of schizophrenia and OCD there are only a few well-controlled studies of the clinical and pathophysiological implications of OC phenomena in schizophrenia, and even these published studies of OC-schizophrenia suffer from design and methodological shortcomings. Although these findings must be verified with controlled studies, evidence suggests that specific symptom assessment and new pharmacological approaches can lead to better clinical outcome in this challenging group of schizophrenia patients. At present, we recommend that clinicians, after careful evaluation of various clinical factors (e.g., clinical course, family history, past treatment response, presence or absence of other coexisting psychiatric and medical conditions), consider adding an adjunctive SSRI or clomipramine therapy along with antipsychotics for at least selective schizophrenia patients with prominent OC features.

References

Allen L, Tejera C: Treatment of clozapine induced obsessive-compulsive symptoms with sertraline (letter). Am J Psychiatry 151:1096–1097, 1994

American Psychiatric Association: Diagnostic and Statistical Manual of Mental Disorders, 4th Edition. Washington, DC, American Psychiatric Association, 1994

Baker RW, Bermanzohn PC, Wirsching DA, et al: Obsessions, compulsions clozapine and risperidone. CNS Spectrums 2(3):26–36, 1997

Bark N, Lindenmayer JP: Ineffectiveness of clomipramine for obsessive-compulsive symptoms in patients with schizophrenia (letter). Am J Psychiatry 149:136–137, 1992

Berman I, Kalinowski A, Berman SM, et al: Obsessive and compulsive symptoms in chronic schizophrenia. Compr Psychiatry 36:6–10, 1995

Berman I, Pappas D, Berman S: Obsessive-compulsive symptoms in schizophrenia: are they manifestations of a distinct subclass of schizophrenia? CNS Spectrums 2(3):45–48, 1997

Bermanzohn PC, Porto L, Arlow PB, et al: Obsessions and delusions: separate and distinct or overlapping? CNS Spectrums 2(3):58–61, 1997

Bermanzohn PC, Porto L, Siris SG, et al: Hierarchical diagnosis in schizophrenia: clinical study of co-occurring syndromes. Schizophr Bull 26:519–527, 2000

Bland RC, Newman SC, Orn H: Schizophrenia: lifetime comorbidity in a community sample. Acta Psychiatr Scand 75:383–391, 1987

Bleuler E: Dementia Praecox, or the Group of Schizophrenias (1911). Translated by Zinken J. New York, International Universities Press, 1950

Bumke O: Lehrbuch der Geisteskrankheiten, 3rd Edition. Munchen, Bergmann, 1944

Butler RW, Jenkins MA, Sprock J, et al: Wisconsin Card Sort Test deficits in chronic paranoid schizophrenia. Schizophr Res 7:169–176, 1992

Ciraulo DA, Shader RI: Fluoxetine drug-drug interactions, I: antidepressant and antipsychotics. J Clin Psychopharmacol 10:48–50, 1990

Eisen JL, Beer DA, Pato MT, et al: Obsessive-compulsive disorder in patients with schizophrenia or schizoaffective disorder. Am J Psychiatry 154:271–273, 1997

Fenton WS, McGlashan TH: The prognostic significance of obsessive-compulsive symptoms in schizophrenia. Am J Psychiatry 143:437–441, 1986

Foa EB, Kozak MJ: DSM-IV field trial: obsessive-compulsive disorder. Am J Psychiatry 152:90–96, 1995

Freud A: Obsessional neurosis: a summary of psychoanalytic views as presented at the congress. Int J Psychoanal 47:116–122, 1966

Freud S: Further recommendations in the technique of psychoanalysis (1908), in The Standard Edition of the Complete Psychological Works of Sigmund Freud, Vol 2. Translated and edited by Strachey J. London, Hogarth Press, 1957, pp 342–365

Ghaemi SN, Pope HG: Lack of insight in psychotic and affective disorders: a review of empirical studies. Harv Rev Psychiatry 2:22–33, 1994

Ghaemi SN, Zarate CA, Popli AP, et al: Is there relationship between clozapine and obsessive compulsive disorder? A retrospective chart review. Compr Psychiatry 36:267–270, 1995

Goff DC, Midha KK, Brotman AW, et al: Elevation of plasma concentration of haloperidol after the addition of fluoxetine. Am J Psychiatry 148:790–792, 1991

Greist JH, Jefferson JW, Kobak KA, et al: Efficacy and tolerability of serotonin transport inhibitors in obsessive-compulsive disorder: a meta-analysis. Arch Gen Psychiatry 52:53–60, 1995

Hollander E (ed): Obsessive-Compulsive–Related Disorders. Washington, DC, American Psychiatric Press, 1993

Hwang MY, Hollander E: Schizophrenia with obsessive-compulsive features: clinical and neuropsychological study. Poster presentation at the annual meeting of the American College of Neuropsychopharmacology, San Juan, Puerto Rico, December 1992

Hwang MY, Opler LA: Schizophrenia with obsessive-compulsive features: assessment and treatment. Psychiatric Annals 24:468–472, 1994

Hwang MY, Opler LA: Management of schizophrenia with obsessive-compulsive disorder. Psychiatric Annals 30:23–28, 2000

Hwang MY, Martin AM, Lindenmayer JP, et al: Treatment of schizophrenia with obsessive-compulsive features with serotonin reuptake inhibitors (letter). Am J Psychiatry 150:1127, 1993

Hwang MY, Rho J, Opler LA, et al: Treatment of obsessive-compulsive schizophrenic patient with clomipramine: clinical and neuropsychological findings. Neuropsychiatry Neuropsychol Behav Neurol 8:231–233, 1995

Hwang MY, Morgan JE, Losonczy MF: Clinical and neuropsychological profiles of OC schizophrenia. J Neuropsychiatry Clin Neurosci 12:91–94, 2000

Insel TR, Akiskal HS: Obsessive-compulsive disorder with psychotic features: a phenomenologic analysis. Am J Psychiatry 143:1527–1533, 1986

Jahrreiss W: Obsessions during schizophrenia. Archiv für Psychiatrie 77:740–788, 1926

Karno M, Golding JM, Sorenson SB, et al: The epidemiology of obsessive-compulsive disorder in five U.S. communities. Arch Gen Psychiatry 45:1094–1099, 1988

Kendler KS, Glazer WM, Morgenstern H: Dimensions of delusional experience. Am J Psychiatry 140:466–469, 1983

Lindenmayer JP, Vakharia M, Kanofsky D: Fluoxetine in chronic schizophrenia (letter). J Clin Psychopharmacol 10:76, 1990

McDougle CJ, Fleischmann RL, Epperson CN, et al: Risperidone addition in fluvoxamine refractory obsessive-compulsive disorder: three cases. J Clin Psychiatry 56:526–528, 1995

Meghani SR, Penick EC, Nickel EJ, et al: Schizophrenia patients with and without OCD (NR138), in 1998 New Research Program and Abstracts, American Psychiatric Association Annual Meeting, Toronto, Ontario, Canada, May 1998. Washington, DC, American Psychiatric Association, 1998

Opler LA, Ramirez PM, Rosenkilde CE, et al: Neurocognitive features of chronic schizophrenic patients. J Nerv Ment Disord 179:638–640, 1991

Patel B, Tandon R: Development of obsessive-compulsive symptoms during clozapine treatment (letter). Am J Psychiatry 150:836, 1993

Porto L, Bermanzohn PC, Pollack S, et al: A profile of obsessive-compulsive symptoms in schizophrenia. CNS Spectrums 2(3):26–33, 1997

Pulman J, Yassa R, Ananth J: Clomipramine treatment of repetitive behavior. Can J Psychiatry 29:254–255, 1984

Regier DA, Boyd JH, Burke JD, et al: One month prevalence of mental disorders in the United States. Arch Gen Psychiatry 45:977–986, 1988

Rosen I: The clinical significance of obsessions in schizophrenia. Journal of Mental Science 103:778–785, 1957

Samuels J, Nestadt G, Wolyniec P, et al: Obsessive-compulsive symptoms in schizophrenia (abstract). Schizophr Res 9:139, 1993

Sasson Y, Bermanzohn PC, Zohar J: Treatment of obsessive-compulsive syndromes in schizophrenia. CNS Spectrums 2(4):34–45, 1997

Siris SG: Adjunctive medication in the maintenance treatment of schizophrenia and its conceptual implications. Br J Psychiatry 163(suppl 22):66–78, 1993

Solyom L, DiNicola VF, Sookman D, et al: Is there an obsessive psychosis? Aetiological and prognostic factors of an atypical form of obsessive compulsive neurosis. Can J Psychiatry 30:372–379, 1985

Spitzer M: On defining delusions. Compr Psychiatry 31:377–379, 1985

Stengel E: A study on some clinical aspects of the relationship between obsessional neurosis and psychotic reaction types. Journal of Mental Science 91:166–184, 1945

Stoll AL, Tohen M, Baldessarini R: Increasing frequency of the diagnosis of obsessive compulsive disorder. Am J Psychiatry 149:638–640, 1992

Stroebel CF, Szarek BL, Grueck BC: Use of clomipramine in treatment of obsessive-compulsive symptomatology. J Clin Psychopharmacol 4:98–100, 1984

Westphal K: Über Zwangsvorstellungen. Archiv für Psychiatrie und Nervenkrankheiten 8:734–750, 1878

Yaryura-Tobias JA, Neziroglu MA, Bergman L: Clomipramine for O-C neurosis: an organic approach. Current Therapuetics Research 20:541–548, 1976

Zohar J: Is there room for another diagnostic subtype—the schizoobsessive subtype? (editorial) CNS Spectrums 2(3):49–50, 1997

Zohar J, Kaplan Z, Benjamin J: Clomipramine treatment of obsessive compulsive symptomatology in schizophrenic patients. J Clin Psychiatry 54:385–388, 1993

CHAPTER 4

Panic Symptoms in Patients With Schizophrenia

Richard J. Pitch, M.D.
Paul C. Bermanzohn, M.D.
Samuel G. Siris, M.D.

Anxiety and even terror are well known to occur prominently in some patients with schizophrenia. Sometimes, these conditions present phenomenologically as a panic attack. Some schizophrenia patients even meet the full criteria for panic disorder. However, panic syndromes associated with schizophrenia only recently have begun to be studied.

The concept of associated psychiatric syndromes (APS) in patients with schizophrenia, as discussed in Chapter 1 of this volume, is productive for understanding complicated cases and improving treatment. Panic is a common psychiatric syndrome that can be considered an APS in schizophrenia. In this chapter, we explore the evidence that panic symptoms occur commonly in patients with schizophrenia and that standard antipanic treatments may benefit these patients. Factors that, in the past, interfered with the recognition of panic in this patient group are identified. In addition, we explore the relationship between panic and paranoia. These observations could have practical implications for diagnosis and treatment.

Definitions and Diagnostic Criteria

The essential feature of a panic attack is a discrete period of intense fear or discomfort that is accompanied by cognitive or somatic symptoms. The cognitive symptoms include derealization or depersonalization, fear of losing control or going crazy, and fear of impending catastrophe or dying. The somatic symptoms include palpitations or tachycardia, sweating, shortness of breath, choking or smothering sensations, chest pain, nausea, dizziness or lightheadedness, parasthesias, and chills or hot flushes. Four or more of these accompanying symptoms must be present to meet the criteria for a panic attack.

Since panic attacks occur in the context of a variety of disorders, DSM-IV (American Psychiatric Association 1994) does not consider "panic attack" to be a codable disorder. To meet the DSM-IV criteria for panic disorder, additional criteria must be met. Panic attacks must be recurrent, but the threshold quantity that counts as "recurrent" is not specified in DSM-IV as it was in DSM-III-R. Some of the panic attacks must be "unexpected." They cannot be restricted to certain situational cues (i.e., public speaking in social phobia, or heights, elevators, or insects in specific phobias), which would then make them better explained by another disorder. Some may argue that all panic attacks are cued by something, whether internal or external, conscious or unconscious, and therefore are never spontaneous. However, the DSM-IV term "unexpected" gets around this by implying that the attack *feels* spontaneous to the patient.

The patient must have persistent concern about having additional attacks, worry about the implication or consequences of the attacks, or undergo a significant behavioral change related to the attacks. Criterion B of panic disorder simply separates two disorders by the presence or absence of agoraphobia. The rest of the criteria serve to exclude panic attacks caused by substances, medical conditions, or other mental disorders. Note that the presence of schizophrenia does not disqualify a diagnosis of panic disorder.

Anxiety and fear are both defined as feelings of apprehension caused by the anticipation of danger, which may be internal or external. Anxiety, however, is a response to a threat that is vague or unknown, whereas fear is a response to a known danger. From a cognitive-processing model (Beck and Emory 1985), pathological anxiety results from faulty, distorted, or counterproductive thinking patterns, in which a person either overestimates the degree of danger and probability of harm or underestimates his or her ability to cope with the perceived threat. Put another way, pathological anxiety can be viewed as an impairment in reality testing. The threat is not really as serious as it feels. Some individuals maintain an awareness of that fact and experience their anxiety as unwarranted (ego-dystonic), though distressing. Others begin to lose that awareness and become harder to reassure. Somewhere along the line of this distortion of reality and loss of reality testing we define the phenomenon of a *delusion*, which is a false, fixed belief. A persecutory delusion is a false, fixed belief that one is being or going to be harmed. The person clings to the belief despite significant evidence against it. Thus, a spectrum from excessive unrealistic worry to frankly delusional thinking becomes evident.

Clinical Relevance

Why is it important to recognize and treat panic syndromes in patients with schizophrenia? In his analysis of Epidemiologic Catchment Area (ECA) data, Boyd (1986) pointed out that panic attacks bring more people into treatment than any other mental disorder and that people with panic disorder are very heavy users of mental health services. Panic disorder is associated with suicide attempts, alcohol abuse, depression, social impairment, financial dependence, and visits to the emergency room (Markowitz et al. 1989). Among patients with schizophrenia or schizoaffective disorder and postpsychotic depression, a lifetime history of panic attacks or panic disorder was found to be associated with a history of suicidal ideation (Siris et al. 1993). Schizophrenia patients are already at increased risk for these problems.

Panic disorder is also a treatable condition, with a number of pharmacological and nonpharmacological strategies available (Coplan et al. 1996). A large literature substantiates this in nonschizophrenia patients with panic disorder.

Several important questions arise, then. How common is it for schizophrenia patients to have significant panic symptoms? Are the available antipanic treatments beneficial and safe for patients with schizophrenia? What impact will these treatments have on their panic symptoms, their symptoms of schizophrenia, and their levels of functioning? What impact will these treatments have on the mental health services system, in which cost and limited resources are of increasing concern?

Epidemiology of Panic in Patients With Schizophrenia

Although the literature is sparse, those reports that have examined the issue have found that panic attacks occur commonly in patients with schizophrenia. The largest scale prevalence study of panic attacks occurring in patients with schizophrenia used ECA data. This program involved five large community samples (total $N = 18,572$). Reviewing those data, Boyd (1986) found that 28%–63% of subjects with schizophrenia reported panic attacks, depending on the community. It should be noted that Boyd specified panic attacks, not full panic disorder, which has stricter criteria and and so probably was less prevalent. Diagnoses were established with the NIMH Diagnostic Interview Schedule (DIS), a structured interview designed to be conducted by lay interviewers, in this case coded to approximate DSM-III (American Psychiatric Association 1980) diagnoses. Because of the possible discrepancies between DIS diagnoses and clinical diagnoses, Boyd was careful to label the diagnoses in the study as DIS disorders rather than DSM-III disorders.

Examining the same ECA data, Tien and Eaton (1992) found that panic attacks were associated with increased odds (relative risk = 2.28) of developing schizophrenia by the reassessment interview 1 year later. This, however, was a relationship that did not achieve statistical significance (P = 0.062).

Argyle (1990) reported on 20 consecutive patients attending an outpatient clinic for maintenance treatment of chronic schizophrenia. Seven of these patients (35%) had regularly occurring panic attacks, and Argyle described each case. Diagnoses were established from ICD-9 criteria and the Structured Clinical Interview for DSM-III-R. Four of the 7 patients (18%) met the full criteria for panic disorder. He found agoraphobia in 3 of the patients with panic attacks and in 1 without panic. Among the 13 patients with significant social avoidance, 4 (20% of the total sample) had typical social phobia, with fears of appearing anxious and being humiliated.

Cutler and Siris (1991) reported on a series of 45 patients, mostly outpatients, with Research Diagnostic Criteria (RDC)—defined schizophrenia or schizoaffective disorder who also had operationally defined postpsychotic depression. Eleven of these patients (24%) had panic attacks as defined by RDC criteria. The authors did not report on the number of patients who met the full criteria for panic disorder. One might at first attribute this high prevalence rate to the fact that these were depressed patients, since the rate of panic attacks is much higher in nonschizophrenia patients with major depression (15%–30%) than in the general population (1%–2%) (Boyd 1986; Grunhaus 1988; Robins et al. 1984). However, in this study, panic patients could not be distinguished by their degree of depression on measures of the Schedule for Affective Disorders and Schizophrenia or the Brief Psychiatric Rating Scale (BPRS) instruments. Panic patients also were not distributed unevenly by other features, such as severity of delusions, hallucinations, thought disorder, negative symptoms, or drug or alcohol abuse.

In these epidemiological studies of panic in patients with schizophrenia, nothing has been written about gender or ethnicity that distinguishes it from panic in the absence of schizophrenia.

Bermanzohn et al. (1995, 2000) are investigating the prevalence of APS in patients with chronic schizophrenia attending a continuing day treatment program. Data on the first 37 patients have been presented. Four patients (10.8%) met the full criteria for panic disorder; two of these patients met the criteria for panic disorder with agoraphobia.

A number of factors have made it difficult for clinicians and investigators to recognize panic in schizophrenia patients. The first factor is diagnostic reductionism. Hierarchical concepts are imbedded in our diagnostic system, probably based on the belief that each patient may have only one diagnosis (Boyd et al. 1984). This belief is rooted in a medical tradition that has been traced back to the 17th century (Boyd et al. 1984; Foucault 1975). Such hierarchical concepts were formalized in psychiatric nosology in DSM-III, where many psychiatric disorders, panic disorder among them, could not be diagnosed if they were "due to" another disorder (e.g., schizophrenia). It was left unclear how to determine that one disorder was due to another. Since anxiety symptoms were thought to be due to schizophrenia, anxiety disorders were generally not diagnosed when a patient had already received a diagnosis of schizophrenia. Many clinicians attach little diagnostic importance to the fact that their schizophrenia patient is very anxious, because "who wouldn't be anxious if they thought they were being followed by the CIA?" In this way a panic disorder might be explained away by, absorbed into, or reduced to the schizophrenia (see Chapter 1, this volume, for a more detailed discussion of diagnostic reductionism). Second, schizophrenia patients may not reveal their panic symptoms because of shame or fear of being hospitalized (Bermanzohn et al. 1995). Third, the way schizophrenia patients do present their panic symptoms may be intertwined with psychotic symptoms or confused with other causes of anxiety.

Patient Assessment and Differential Diagnosis

The nature of the panic attacks, as well as the associated anticipatory anxiety and avoidance behaviors, seems to be virtually identical to those symptoms reported by patients without schizophrenia (Cutler 1994). However, patients with schizophrenia frequently communicate in odd or ineffective ways, which could make it difficult to recognize a panic syndrome. In addition, schizophrenia patients frequently present their panic symptoms with a psychotic overlay, explaining them with or incorporating them into delusional material (Cutler 1994; Kahn et al. 1988). Panic attacks may even be associated with an actual increase in delusions and hallucinations (Cutler 1994; Cutler and Siris 1991).

When panic symptoms are intertwined with psychotic ones, the somatic symptoms associated with panic attacks may provide specific clues:

> Ms. S. is a 35-year-old unemployed single woman who lives with her parents. She has a 15-year history of chronic paranoid schizophrenia with persecutory and referential delusions and auditory hallucinations. These delusions and hallucinations have been almost continuous throughout her illness and refractory to multiple neuroleptics.
>
> For the past several years, she also has had panic attacks, sometimes unexpectedly but usually confined to the evenings or waking her up during the night. Typically, she describes episodic intense fear that her parents are dead or will be harmed. This is accompanied by palpitations, sweating, shortness of breath, feelings of being smothered, choking sensations, and derealization. She worries that if they are dead, she will be all alone and unable to take care of herself. She also is sure that she would be accused of murdering them and that, because of her schizophrenia history, no one would believe her innocence. She thinks she would be confined in either a jail or a state hospital for the rest of her life. Her panic symptoms progress in intensity, usually until she checks their room to see if they are breathing, at which point she usually feels reassured. Because these attacks occur almost every night, she delays going to sleep and has difficulty falling asleep, fearing both the attack itself and the sensation of being alone.

Patients with schizophrenia can also present with other anxiety syndromes in the course of the illness that must be distinguished from panic syndromes. The differential diagnosis includes prodromal anxiety, social phobia, agoraphobia, akathisia, medical conditions, and substance-related anxiety (Table 4–1). In prodromal anxiety, patients may report a free-floating anxiety or a hypervigilance that they cannot explain before going on to develop frank psychotic symptoms. Like depression, anxiety is sometimes an early manifestation of a psychotic relapse (Docherty et al. 1978). Anxiety and agitation can also arise as a component of increased psychosis. Patients may become hypervigilant (e.g., as a natural response to delusions of persecution or thought broadcasting), become fearful of losing control to dangerous command hallucinations, or anticipate confinement from the experience of prior hospitalizations. This is the kind of anxiety that may be more appropriately subsumed into the syndrome of schizophrenia, in contrast to other manifestations of anxiety that warrant additional diagnoses.

Patients with schizophrenia may have difficulty negotiating the intricate and subtle rules of social interaction, and this difficulty provokes and is maintained by anxiety in social situations. "Social anxiety" usually implies the fear of being embarrassed in front of others. Social phobia is another diagnostic entity characterized by marked and persistent fear of

Table 4–1. Differential diagnosis of anxiety in patients with schizophrenia

Prodromal anxiety
Anxiety as part of the psychosis
Social skills deficits
Social anxiety, social phobia
Agoraphobia
Panic attacks, panic disorder
Akathisia
Medication side effects
Medical conditions
Substances of abuse (including caffeine and nicotine)

social situations in which embarrassment may occur, associated with social avoidance or dread, recognition that the fear is excessive, and acute anxiety responses in social situations (which can take the form of panic attacks). This disorder, as well as agoraphobia, is enormously difficult to recognize in patients with schizophrenia, because phenotypically it can resemble paranoia or negative symptoms. Social isolation in patients with schizophrenia often has been attributed to deficits in social skills, but social anxiety may also be a significant contributor to this problem (Penn et al. 1994). Establishing why a patient avoids certain situations is critical (Mannuzza et al. 1986). Patients with panic disorder might say they fear primarily that people will notice that they are having a panic attack, whereas people with social phobia fear embarrassment from the social exposure:

> Mrs. M. is a 49-year-old divorced psychologist with late-onset chronic paranoid schizophrenia, now with prominent negative symptoms but originally with complex paranoid and bizarre delusions. She had a history of panic disorder with agoraphobia that preceded the onset of her schizophrenia by more than 10 years. The panic disorder was complicated by alcohol abuse, now in remission for 1 year.
>
> Mrs. M. presented to a partial hospital program with chief complaints of anhedonia, lack of spontaneity, and poverty of thought, as well as an inability to travel on public transportation, which limited her access to desirable activities. On admission, she described limited-symptom attacks, consisting of episodic fear of "becoming sick again" associated with palpitations, lightheadedness, and the urge to escape. She would worry at those times about being hospitalized. These episodes occured primarily on exposure to public transportation but also occasionally occurred unexpectedly. Mrs. M. also displayed significant parkinsonian symptoms, including bradyphrenia, bradykinesia, masked facies, and flat

affect that was difficult to tease out from the deficit symptoms of schizophrenia. She had no active delusions, hallucinations, or formal thought disorder. Mrs. M. was not dysphoric, and she lacked vegetative signs of depression. She was taking molindone 50 mg po hs but no other medications.

In the partial hospital, lorazepam 1.5 mg/day was added, and she received supportive and cognitive therapies in groups and individually. Her panic symptoms were completely eliminated within 2 weeks. By the third week, she was able to travel independently on the bus. The molindone was then lowered to 25 mg hs, with some improvement in spontaneity and motivation. Her affective display and movements also became more supple.

Akathisia is an extrapyramidal syndrome produced by antipsychotic and possibly other medications that can present as a phenocopy of anxiety (Van Putten 1975). Patients experience a sense of muscular tension or motor restlessness; they appear fidgety and sometimes pace or "march in place." This motor symptom is often hard to distinguish from psychic anxiety, psychotic agitation, or agitated depression. A large number of medications can produce anxiety as a side effect, and many medical conditions can produce anxiety syndromes (e.g., arrhythmias, hypoglycemia, hyperthyroidism). It is important to remember that schizophrenia patients may also become medically ill; clinical leads must be followed so that these medical conditions can be treated. Finally, substances of abuse, including caffeine and nicotine, frequently cause anxiety symptoms during either intoxication or withdrawal from the substance. Patients with schizophrenia are at increased risk for substance abuse as well as interactions from polypharmacy, which should be considered in the differential diagnosis and treatment of anxiety in this population (see Chapter 7, this volume).

Etiological Considerations

The interaction between panic symptoms and psychosis requires further understanding. A stress-diathesis model has been proposed for psychosis in schizophrenia (Neuchterlein and Dawson 1984; Zubin and Spring 1977). In that model, various stressors can provoke or exacerbate psychotic symptoms in vulnerable individuals. Theoretically, panic attacks could also act as endogenous stressors (Siris 1988, 1993). In patients with schizophrenia who also have panic symptoms, the two diatheses may interact in a dynamic way, creating a vicious cycle of symptoms. Particularly when patients describe their panic symptoms with psychotic terms, the panic can be confused with symptoms of schizophrenia, especially paranoia.

Mr. C. is a 22-year-old single man who had carried a diagnosis of chronic paranoid schizophrenia for 5 years. When he came to a partial hospital program, his diagnosis was changed to psychotic disorder not otherwise specified because on careful reassessment the only "A" criterion in his history was frequent delusions of persecution and reference. He also met the full criteria for panic disorder, obsessive-compulsive disorder, and a severe schizotypal personality.

Mr. C. had spontaneous panic attacks but was especially vulnerable to them whenever he went out of the house, particularly into crowded situations. He was exquisitely sensitive to other people glancing at him and would believe that they considered him "weird" or "feminine." He would become angry that they were judging him. Often, he would then become fearful, with palpitations, sweating, muscular tension, dry mouth, and lightheadedness. He would become unable to concentrate at all, feeling like his thoughts were "blocked." He labeled these episodes "phase outs," and it took several interviews before the entire panic syndrome was elicited.

Mr. C. stated he feels very uncomfortable around crowds of people because he fears they will stare at him and make him "paranoid," and he fears he will act on violent thoughts in response to that. In trying to tease out the panic symptoms from the difficulties in reality testing, he said, "I just can't tell where the paranoia ends and the anxiety begins. They feel the same, all mixed together."

Klein (1980) has noted that before panic disorder was described as a separate entity, patients with what we now call panic disorder were often diagnosed with schizophrenia.

Patients with schizophrenia may be at increased risk for anxiety because of their misinterpretations of danger or, sometimes, because of their own appreciation of their impaired coping strategies. When they are unable to filter out environmental stimuli as insignificant, they may experience stereotypic ideas of reference or persecution and become hypervigilant and fearful. In schizophrenia patients with panic disorder, these cues can contribute to increasingly heightened anxiety and autonomic discharge, leading to a full-blown panic attack. With repeated events, the person may become progressively hypervigilant of the warning signs and eventually learn more global avoidance behaviors to reduce the risk of the experience happening again. If this occurs, then cognitive retraining, in vivo exposure, and medication might all help the patient to break this vicious cycle and learn more adaptive coping strategies, leading to restored functioning.

In a controlled family study, Heun and Maier (1995) examined possible reasons for comorbidity of schizophrenia and panic disorder by analyzing the aggregation patterns of these disorders in first-degree relatives of patients and control subjects. These patterns were then compared with those patterns that would be predicted by various models of comorbidity. Heun and Maier found that the frequency of panic disorder was enhanced in relatives of schizophrenia patients without panic disorder in comparison to control subjects and that the frequencies for panic disorder were equivalent in relatives of patients with schizophrenia, with panic disorder, and with comorbidity. They argued that this pattern did not support a model in which the two disorders are causally linked, such as a stress-diathesis model, in which the presence of one disorder induces the expression of the other. Rather, they suggested that familial vulnerability factors *underlying* schizophrenia might lead to the expression of panic disorder. The reverse was not supported in this sample; that is, the frequency of schizophrenia was not enhanced in relatives of patients with panic disorder.

Some have suggested that panic attacks may be specifically associated with paranoia. In a reassessment of the ECA study data (P. C. Bermanzohn et al., unpublished data, 1996), schizophrenic persons with panic attacks were almost 3 times more likely to also have paranoia than were schizophrenic persons without panic symptoms. Among individuals who do not have schizophrenia, the chance of having paranoia was about 10 times greater if they had panic attacks than if they did not have panic attacks. Neenan et al. (1986) described two patients with chronic panic disorder and no difficulties with socialization before their illness who showed pronounced schizoid, paranoid, and schizotypal traits on standard personality tests. These investigators later found significant paranoid personality traits in 15 of 28 outpatients (54%) with panic disorder (Reich and Braginsky 1994). They suggested that social withdrawal due to years of suffering from panic disorder potentially could result in the development of these personality traits.

Treatment

In panic disorder patients without schizophrenia, a number of pharmacological treatments are available. Imipramine and alprazolam are the best substantiated by controlled studies (Ballenger et al. 1988; Cross-National Collaborative Panic Study 1992), but other tricyclics, clonazepam, serotonin reuptake inhibitors, monoamine oxidase inhibitors, and valproate also have support in the literature (for review, see Coplan et al. 1996). Specific nonpharmacological therapies, especially cognitive-behavioral therapy, also have wide support (Barlow et al. 1989; Clark et al. 1985, 1994; Craske et al. 1991; Gitlin et al. 1985; Ost and Westling 1995). However, to our knowledge, there are no published double-blind, placebo-controlled studies on the treatment of panic attacks or panic disorder in patients with schizophrenia. Much of what is available in the literature is based on anecdotal reports.

In one prospective study of open adjunctive treatment with alprazolam (Kahn et al. 1987, 1988), seven inpatients were treated for both schizophrenia and panic disorder (both meeting DSM-III criteria, if the exclusionary criteria at the time would have allowed both diagnoses simultaneously). After their neuroleptic doses were held constant for at least 3 weeks, alprazolam was openly added in a standard titration schedule (up to 0.5 to 0.75 mg qid), maintained for 3 weeks, then tapered over 2 weeks and discontinued for 3 weeks. In all seven cases, panic attacks were reduced during alprazolam treatment and increased after its withdrawal. Interestingly, positive and negative symptoms of schizophrenia also improved and worsened along with the severity of panic symptoms. This led the authors to ponder the interrelatedness of the pathophysiologies of panic disorder and schizophrenia.

Similar results were reported in a single case study of a patient with chronic paranoid schizophrenia who also had what the patient himself called "paranoid attacks" (Sandberg and Siris 1987). These attacks consisted of classic panic symptoms, with their cognitive and autonomic somatic components, associated with simultaneous increases in delusions and hallucinations. Various manipulations of the neuroleptic medications offered no benefit. After a stable neuroleptic regimen was maintained, alprazolam 0.5 mg tid was added, and the patient immediately experienced a cessation of these attacks for 3.5 weeks. The attacks did eventually return in an attentuated form. The alprazolam was increased to 5 mg/day, resulting in improvement in both panic and psychotic symptoms as well as in the patient's functioning.

A number of studies have examined the effectiveness of alprazolam for negative symptoms of schizophrenia, with mixed results (Adan and Siris 1989; Csernansky et al. 1984, 1988; Wolkowitz et al. 1986). Since these studies did not specifically examine the patients for the presence of panic attacks, there remains the question of what role, if any, panic played in the cases of successful treatment.

Benzodiazepines have also been studied in schizophrenia in general with mixed results. Siris (1993) suggested that the results might have been more consistant had patients been preselected for the presence of anxiety disorders.

Several treatment strategies were described, with mixed results, in a case series of patients with schizophrenia and panic symptoms (Argyle 1990). When the dose of neuroleptic was increased, panic was relieved in two patients, whereas in two others panic symptoms were exacerbated, even though psychosis and agitation were reduced. Augmentation with diazepam (5 mg bid or 2.5 mg tid) reduced panic in two patients; in another patient, panic improved with alprazolam augmentation (0.5 mg tid).

Yeragani et al. (1989) reported on two cases of patients with residual schizophrenia and comorbid panic attacks consisting of discrete periods of intense anxiety associated with several autonomic symptoms. In both cases, addition of low doses of imipramine (50 mg/day) was followed by "moderate to marked improvement" in the panic attacks, without any change in psychotic symptoms.

Siris et al. (1989) described two more cases in which imipramine was beneficial in the treatment of patients with schizophrenia and panic disorder (defined by DSM-III-R [American Psychiatric Association 1987] criteria). These patients also had significant depressive symtoms. The first patient received placebo (under double-blind conditions) for 9 weeks, without change in symptoms. She then received imipramine 150 mg/day (openly administered) and achieved full remission of her psychotic, depressive, and panic symptoms for the first time in 10 years. After 6 months, the imipramine was discontinued (under double-blind conditions), and all three types of symptoms returned within 1 month. When imipramine was resumed, symptoms in all three spheres (psychotic, depressive, and panic) and social functioning improved again within 2–4 weeks. This A-B-A-B experimental pattern strengthens the suggestion of imipramine's effectiveness. In the second case, the A-B-A-B test pattern was not employed, but imipramine 200 mg/day was administered under double-blind conditions and, as in the first case, resulted in improvement in functioning and reduction of symptoms of panic, depression, and psychosis.

Caution should be used when administering antidepressant medication to patients with schizophrenia. However, this can be done safely and beneficially (for review, see Chapter 2, this volume) by maintaining and adjusting neuroleptic medication, being mindful of drug-drug interactions, and diligently assessing signs and symptoms—all of which are normally part of good patient care.

Pilot data from our group (Arlow et al. 1996) suggest that cognitive-behavioral group therapy with some modifications may be effective. In an open 16-week clinical trial of eight patients who met DSM-III-R criteria for both schizophrenia and panic disorder, panic symptoms were reduced in frequency and intensity posttreatment. There is also one case report in which a patient with chronic schizophrenia complicated by agoraphobia without panic attacks responded favorably to a combination of behavior therapy and diazepam (Finkel 1987).

Thus, although there have been few systematic treatment trials, the data suggest that the modalities used to treat panic without schizophrenia (both pharmacological and cognitive-behavioral) also may be used to treat panic with schizophrenia. More systematic study is needed to demonstrate both the safety and the efficacy of these modalities in this population.

Summary

Data suggest that panic attacks occur in approximately 25% of schizophrenia patients. Full-blown panic disorder probably occurs less often but may occur at a rate higher than in the general population. Schizophrenia is an illness associated with severe disability and suffering. Comorbid panic attacks contribute significantly to the suffering and disability of patients with schizophrenia and may be associated with chronicity in this population. As such, it may be useful to consider panic as an associated psychiatric syndrome in schizophrenia worthy of specific attention. Panic attacks are phenomenologically similar in patients with schizophrenia, as they are in nonschizophrenia patients. However, a number of factors lead clinicians away from recognizing panic syndromes in these patients. Therefore, panic in patients with schizophrenia may be underdiagnosed and, consequently, undertreated.

Probably the most useful course of action now is to reexamine patients with schizophrenia for the presence of associated panic attacks or panic disorder and to give a careful clinical trial of standard antipanic treatments (pharmacological and nonpharmacological) adjunctively with their antipsychotic medication. To date, there are no controlled treatment studies, only a few anecdotal but highly suggestive case reports, and pilot data. However, these early reports, in addition to a larger literature on depression in patients with schizophrenia, support the safety and efficacy of these treatments under carefully monitored circumstances in which antipsychotic medications are used simultaneously. Treating the associated panic also may reduce the severity of both the positive and the negative symptoms of schizophrenia and increase overall functioning. Results from a randomized, double-blind study of adjunctive antipanic medication in schizophrenia patients selected for panic symptoms still need to be published.

References

Adan F, Siris SG: Trials of adjunctive alprazolam in "negative symptom" patients. Can J Psychiatry 34:326–328, 1989

American Psychiatric Association: Diagnostic and Statistical Manual of Mental Disorders, 3rd Edition. Washington, DC, American Psychiatric Association, 1980

American Psychiatric Association: Diagnostic and Statistical Manual of Mental Disorders, 3rd Edition, Revised. Washington, DC, American Psychiatric Association, 1987

American Psychiatric Association: Diagnostic and Statistical Manual of Mental Disorders, 4th Edition. Washington, DC, American Psychiatric Association, 1994

Argyle N: Panic attacks in chronic schizophrenia. Br J Psychiatry 157:430–433, 1990

Arlow PB, Moran ME, Bermanzohn PC, et al: A cognitive-behavioral approach to panic attacks in chronic schizophrenia. Poster presented at the 149th annual meeting of the American Psychiatric Association, New York, May 6, 1996

Ballenger JC, Burrows GD, Dupont RL Jr, et al: Alprazolam in panic disorder and agoraphobia: results from a multicenter trial, I. Efficacy in short-term treatment. Arch Gen Psychiatry 45:413–422, 1988

Barlow DH, Craske MG, Cerny JA, et al: Behavioral treatment of panic disorder. Behavior Therapy 20:261–282, 1989

Beck AT, Emery G: Anxiety Disorders and Phobias. New York, Basic Books, 1985

Bermanzohn PC, Porto L, Siris SG: Associated psychiatric syndromes (APS) in chronic schizophrenia, in Proceedings of the 34th Annual Meeting of the American College of Neuropsychopharmacology, San Juan, Puerto Rico, December 13, 1995

Bermanzohn PC, Porto L, Siris SG, et al: Hierarchical diagnosis in chronic schizophrenia: a clinical study of co-occurring syndromes. Schizophr Bull 26:519–527, 2000

Boyd JH: Use of mental health services for the treatment of panic disorder. Am J Psychiatry 143:1569–1574, 1986

Boyd JH, Burke JD Jr, Gruenberg E, et al: Exclusion criteria of DSM-III: a study of co-occurrence of hierarchy-free syndromes. Arch Gen Psychiatry 41:983–989, 1984

Clark DM, Salkovskis PM, Chalkley AJ: Respiratory control as a treatment for panic attacks. J Behav Ther Exp Psychiatry 16:23–30, 1985

Clark DM, Salkovskis PM, Hackmann A, et al: A comparison of cognitive therapy, applied relaxation and imipramine in the treatment of panic disorder. Br J Psychiatry 164:759–769, 1994

Coplan JD, Pine DS, Papp LA, et al: An algorithm-oriented treatment approach for panic disorder. Psychiatric Annals 26:192–201, 1996

Craske MG, Brown TA, Barlow DH: Behavioral treatment of panic disorder: a two-year follow-up. Behavior Therapy 22:289–304, 1991

Cross-National Collaborative Panic Study, Second Phase Investigators: Drug treatment of panic disorder. Comparative efficacy of alprazolam, imipramine, and placebo. Br J Psychiatry 160:191–202 [discussion: 202–205], 1992

Csernansky JG, Lombrozo L, Gulevich GD, et al: Treatment of negative schizophrenic symptoms with alprazolam: a preliminary open-label study. J Clin Psychopharmacol 4:349–352, 1984

Csernansky JG, Riney SJ, Lombrozo L, et al: Double-blind comparison of alprazolam, diazepam, and placebo for the treatment of negative schizophrenic symptoms. Arch Gen Psychiatry 45:655–659, 1988

Cutler J: Panic attacks and schizophrenia: assessment and treatment. Psychiatric Annals 24:473–476, 1994

Cutler JL, Siris SG: "Panic-like" symptomatology in schizophrenic and schizoaffective patients with postpsychotic depression: observations and implications. Compr Psychiatry 32:465–473, 1991

Docherty JP, van Kammen DP, Siris SG, et al: Stages of onset of acute schizophrenic psychosis. Am J Psychiatry 135:720–726, 1978

Finkel JA: Diazepam in a patient with chronic schizophrenia complicated by agoraphobia. J Clin Psychiatry 48:33–34, 1987

Foucault M: The Birth of the Clinic: An Archeology of Medical Perception. St Paul, Vintage Books, 1975

Gitlin B, Martin J, Shear MK, et al: Behavior therapy for panic disorder. J Nerv Ment Dis 173:742–743, 1985

Grunhaus L: Clinical and psychobiological characteristics of simultaneous panic disorder and major depression Am J Psychiatry 145:1214–1219, 1988

Heun R, Maier W: Relationship of schizophrenia and panic disorder: evidence from a controlled family study. Am J Med Genet 60:127–132, 1995

Kahn JP, Puertollano M, Schane MD, et al: Schizophrenia, panic anxiety, and alprazolam (letter). Am J Psychiatry 144:527–528, 1987

Kahn JP, Puertollano M, Schane MD, et al: Schizophrenia, panic anxiety, and alprazolam. Arch Gen Psychiatry 145:742–744, 1988

Klein DF: Anxiety reconceptualized. Compr Psychiatry 21:411–427, 1980

Mannuzza S, Fyer AJ, Klein DF, et al: Schedule for Affective Disorders and Schizophrenia—Lifetime Version Modified for the Study of Anxiety Disorders (SADS-LA): rationale and conceptual development. J Psychiatr Res 20:317–325, 1986

Markowitz JS, Weissman MM, Ouellette R, et al: Quality of life in panic disorder. Arch Gen Psychiatry 46:984–992, 1989

Neenan P, Felkner J, Reich J: Schizoid personality traits developing secondary to panic disorder. J Nerv Ment Dis 174:483, 1986

Neuchterlein KH, Dawson ME: A heuristic vulnerability/stress model of schizophrenia. Schizophr Bull 10:300–312, 1984

Ost LG, Westling BE: Applied relaxation vs cognitive behavior therapy in the treatment of panic disorder. Behav Res Ther 33:145–158, 1995

Penn DL, Hope DA, Spaulding W, et al: Social anxiety in schizophrenia. Schizophr Res 11:277–284, 1994

Reich J, Braginsky Y: Paranoid personality traits in a panic disordered population: a pilot study. Compr Psychiatry 35:260–264, 1994

Robins LN, Helzer JE, Weissman MM, et al: Lifetime prevalence of specific psychiatric disorders in three sites. Arch Gen Psychiatry 41:949–958, 1984

Sandberg L, Siris SG: Panic disorder in schizophrenia. J Nerv Ment Dis 175:627–628, 1987

Siris SG: Implications of normal brain development for the pathogenesis of schizophrenia (letter). Arch Gen Psychiatry 45:1055, 1988

Siris SG: Adjunctive medication in the maintenance treatment of schizophrenia and
its conceptual implications. Br J Psychiatry 163 (suppl 22):66–78, 1993

Siris SG, Aronson A, Sellew AP: Imipramine-responsive panic-like symptomatology in schizophrenia/schizoaffective disorder. Biol Psychiatry 25:485–488,
1989

Siris SG, Mason SE, Shuwall MA: Histories of substance abuse, panic and suicidal
ideation in schizophrenic patients with histories of post-psychotic depressions.
Prog Neuropsychopharmacol Biol Psychiatry 17:609–617, 1993

Tien AY, Eaton WW: Psychopathologic precursers and sociodemographic risk factors for the schizophrenia syndrome. Arch Gen Psychiatry 49:37–46, 1992

Van Putten T: The many faces of akathisia. Compr Psychiatry 16:43–47, 1975

Wolkowitz OM, Pickar D, Doran AR, et al: Combination alprazolam-neuroleptic
treatment of the positive and negative symptoms of schizophrenia. Am J Psychiatry 143:85–87, 1986

Yeragani NK, Balon R, Pohl R: Schizophrenia, panic attacks, and antidepressants
(letter). Am J Psychiatry 146:279, 1989

Zubin J, Spring B: Vulnerability: a new view of schizophrenia. J Abnorm Psychol 86:
103–126, 1977

CHAPTER 5

Medical and Surgical Illness in Patients With Schizophrenia

John H. Gilmore, M.D.
L. Fredrik Jarskog, M.D.
T. Scott Stroup, M.D., M.P.H.

*M*edical illness is common in patients with schizophrenia and presents a variety of challenges to patients and their physicians. Management of medical illness requires that a patient recognize and report symptoms of medical illness, seek out medical care, cooperate with a diagnostic workup, and comply with what can be a complex treatment regimen. If a medical illness arises in a person who is paranoid, amotivated, and disorganized, this difficult task becomes even harder. In addition to the fundamental problems of recognition and management, there is evidence that medical illness can worsen symptoms of schizophrenia. Often questions of informed consent arise. The importance of these issues is increasingly being recognized (Adler and Griffith 1991; Jeste et al. 1996; Vieweg et al. 1995).

In this chapter, we review the epidemiology of medical illness in patients with schizophrenia. We also review the difficulties associated with the recognition and management of medical illness in this unique patient population. With this background, we then offer suggestions for meeting the challenges that medical illness brings to the care of patients with schizophrenia.

Epidemiology

It has long been debated whether patients with schizophrenia have morbidity and mortality rates higher than those in the general population. Most studies support a mortality rate among patients with schizophrenia that is approximately two times that of the general population, for both males and females (Allebeck and Wistedt 1986; Baldwin 1979; Black 1988; Tsuang and Woolson 1977). Tsuang et al. (1980) found patients with schizophrenia to have their lifetime survival shortened by 9–10 years. There is consensus that suicide represents the largest source of excess mortality in this population (Allebeck 1989). Several studies have found standardized mortality ratio values (number of observed deaths divided by number of expected deaths) for suicide in the range of 3 to 15 (Allebeck and Wistedt 1986; Eastwood et al. 1982; Herrman et al. 1983; Tsuang 1978). Tsuang and Woolson (1978) addressed the question of whether unnatural deaths (suicide, homicide, and accidents) are solely responsible for the excess mortality rates among patients with schizophrenia. In their study, after the effect of unnatural deaths was factored out, approximately a twofold excess in natural deaths remained in patients with schizophrenia. These results were based on relatively small numbers of patients but are supported by data from other investigators (Herrman et al. 1983; Mortensen and Juel 1993). Notably, the number of unnatural deaths appears to decrease after the first 5–10 years of follow-up, although this mortality risk may persist longer in males than in females (Simpson and Tsuang 1996).

The overall increase in natural mortality rates in patients with schizophrenia suggests that certain medical illnesses are more prevalent and/or more lethal in this population. Much research has focused on specific disease associations with schizophrenia. Although there are conflicting findings, these studies have important implications for the clinician, because they can heighten awareness of additional risk for specific categories of medical illness. In addition, positive or negative correlations with a particular illness potentially can provide clues to etiologic mechanisms of schizophrenia.

Several studies have found increased rates of mortality from ischemic heart disease in patients with schizophrenia (Allebeck and Wistedt 1986; Hayward 1995; Herrman et al. 1983; Mortensen and Juel 1993; but see Black et al. 1985). The Oxford Record Linkage Study, a study of more than 2 million people since 1963, found that cardiovascular disease was the most common cause of death and accounted for most of the excess mortality in patients with schizophrenia, in both males and females (Herrman et al. 1983). It remains unclear whether the increased mortality due to cardiovascular disease is secondary to schizophrenia itself. The increase in mortality is quite likely due, at least in part, to other variables, including the effects of neuroleptic medications, rates of smoking, and the overall level of physical activity of patients with schizophrenia. The stress of having a psychotic illness may contribute not only to cardiovascular disease but to other diseases as well. Stress has well-documented negative effects on overall physical health and the immune system (Dorian and Garfinkel 1987).

It has long been suggested that patients with schizophrenia have low rates of cancer (for review, see Allebeck 1989), though several studies have found overall cancer mortality rates in patients with schizophrenia to be similar to those in the general population (Baldwin 1980; Craig and Lin 1981; Tsuang et al. 1980). Recently, Mortensen (1994) found, in a study of 9,156 inpatients with schizophrenia in Denmark, that the overall incidence of cancer was reduced. Although the incidence of cancer was reduced, the cancer mortality rate in this group was not statistically different from that in the general population (Mortensen and Juel 1993). Since cancer mortality encompasses cancer incidence as well as survival time and mortality from other illnesses, the use of cancer mortality data in establishing cancer risk has limitations (Mortensen 1994).

Because of the heterogeneity of cancer, identifying associations between the rates of specific types of cancers and schizophrenia may be more relevant. Decreased and increased rates of various subtypes of malignancies have been observed in patients with schizophrenia (Baldwin 1979; Harris 1988; Simpson 1988). Unfortunately, most studies have insufficient sample sizes to detect true associations. Some of the more consistent findings include a reduced risk of lung cancer (Soni and Gill 1979; Tsuang et al. 1983) and an increased risk of breast cancer in females (Baldwin 1979; Ettigi et al. 1973; Masterson and O'Shea 1984; but see Brugmans et al. 1973; Mortensen 1994). A variable that still needs further evaluation is the putative antineoplastic effect of neuroleptics (Driscoll et al. 1978). Since phenothiazines are concentrated in the lungs, the negative trend between lung cancer and schizophrenia could be unrelated to the biological process of schizophrenia. Similarly, the positive association with breast cancer could be related to elevations in serum prolactin levels produced by phenothiazines (Ettigi et al. 1973).

Significant excess mortality from pneumonia has been seen in some studies of populations with schizophrenia (Baldwin 1980; Mortensen and Juel 1993; Tsuang et al. 1980) but not in others (Allebeck and Wistedt 1986). High rates of mortality from infectious diseases in general, including tuberculosis, were frequently reported up until the 1940s (for review, see Baldwin 1979), but these rates were characteristic of institutionalization and were not specifically linked to schizophrenia. It may be that high rates of smoking in patients with schizophrenia contribute to the increased rate of pneumonia (Masterson and O'Shea 1984; Mortensen and Juel 1993). The prevalence of human immunodeficiency virus (HIV) infection is increased among patients with psychiatric illness (Stefan and Catalan 1995), and patients with schizophrenia are particularly at risk (Cournos et al. 1994).

In contrast to most other disease associations with schizophrenia, there appears to be considerable consensus in studies showing a reduced incidence of rheumatoid arthritis. Gregg (1939) found a morbidity rate for arthritis 17 times greater in the general population than among more than 15,000 patients with psychoses (see also Pilkington 1955). More recent studies have used radiographic evidence to confirm the diagnosis of rheumatoid arthritis, and the negative association has remained strong (Allebeck et al. 1985; Baldwin 1980; Harris 1988; Vinogradov et al. 1991). Mechanisms that could explain the negative association include altered prostaglandin metabolism, histocompatibility factors, β-endorphin levels, and altered tryptophan and serotonin metabolism (Vinogradov et al. 1991). Although no clear reason has been discovered to explain the observed relationship, further research in this area could yield etiologic clues for both disorders.

Associations between schizophrenia and reduced rates of cerebrovascular disease (Masterson and O'Shea 1984; but see Baldwin 1980), decreased rates of peptic ulcer disease (Gosling 1958; but see Hussar 1968), and reduced incidence of asthma and other allergic conditions (Ehrentheil 1957; but see Matthysse and Lipinski 1975) have been documented. However, the studies are too small and/or the findings are too conflicting to draw general conclusions.

Patient Assessment and Related Issues

Associations of schizophrenia with specific medical illnesses aside, people with severe mental illness do have a high prevalence of medical disorders (25%–57%), a large percentage of which are unrecognized by health professionals (Barnes et al. 1983; D'Ercole et al. 1991; Koran et al. 1989; Koranyi 1979; McCarrick et al. 1986). Among 529 public psychiatric patients in California, Koran et al. (1989) found that 39% had medical disorders but that the state mental health system had identified only 47% of those illnesses. Patients in state hospitals were particularly at risk for unrecognized medical illnesses. In a study of more than 2,000 persons newly referred to a psychiatric clinic in Canada, Koranyi (1979) found that referring psychiatrists missed medical diagnoses in 48% of the patients, while other physicians missed medical illnesses in 32%.

Patient-related factors are one reason for the high rate of undiagnosed physical disorders. Positive symptoms, negative symptoms, neurocognitive abnormalities, and altered pain thresholds (discussed below) clearly interfere with symptom recognition, symptom reporting, and help seeking. A lack of assertiveness in medical encounters has also been cited as a factor contributing to poor recognition of medical illness in patients with schizophrenia (Lieberman and Coburn 1986). Low socioeconomic status, common among persons with schizophrenia, is a risk factor for many illnesses and may contribute both to the high prevalence of medical disorders and to poor access to health care services (Karasu et al. 1980).

Provider-related issues also contribute to underdiagnosis of medical problems in persons with severe mental illness. Sox et al. (1989) cite the limited physical assessment skills of psychiatric personnel as an important reason for poor recognition. Others suggest that psychiatrists have little interest in medical problems and that they do not feel competent to evaluate or treat nonpsychiatric illnesses (D'Ercole et al. 1991; Lieberman and Coburn 1986). Reasons for this low interest include a belief that others have greater physical examination skills, that physical exams have a low yield, and that physical exams interfere with transference. Particularly at risk are women, because physicians may hesitate to conduct gynecological exams of mentally ill persons for a variety of legal, transference, and countertransference reasons (D'Ercole et al. 1991).

The stigma of mental illness and countertransference issues also contribute to poor medical care for patients with schizophrenia (Vieweg et al. 1995). Stigma, defined by Goffman (1963) as an undesired and discrediting attribute that can lead to discrimination, has long been assigned to people with mental illness (Dain 1994). Societal biases extend to the health care system, placing people with mental illness at risk for poor service from health care providers (Lieberman and Coburn 1986). All types of physicians are subject to countertransference problems with frightening, noncompliant, or unhygienic patients. Patients with "imaginary" voices and bizarre beliefs may be assumed to have imagined medical problems. The result is that patients with schizophrenia may get poorer evaluations and treatments (Lieberman and Coburn 1986).

Systemic problems also contribute to inadequate recognition of medical illnesses in a variety of ways. Fragmentation of medical and psychiatric services in community settings, where the vast majority of patients with schizophrenia now live, makes coordinated care difficult (Lieberman and Coburn 1986). Psychiatric clinics and inpatient units often lack facilities to conduct medical evaluations (D'Ercole et al. 1991). Inadequate financial and social support for persons with mental disabilities leaves them with risk factors for medical illness and limited access to health care services.

Because Medicaid is an important payer for medical care for persons with disabilities in the United States, complex eligibility requirements limit access to medical care for persons with severe mental illness (Lieberman and Coburn 1986). The rapid conversion of state Medicaid programs into managed systems of care may exacerbate problems in the coordination of medical and psychiatric care. Although managed care plans in the United States often use primary care physicians as coordinators of all health care services to improve accountability, the trend of "carving out" mental health services to behavioral health managed care networks may undermine this advantage (Stroup and Dorwart 1997).

Symptoms Associated With Schizophrenia That Interfere With Medical Care

A variety of other factors can interfere with a patient's ability to live a healthy lifestyle, detect and report symptoms of medical illness, or engage in and comply with treatment. These factors include the major symptoms of schizophrenia itself, as well as the related phenomena of poor insight, poor compliance, and altered pain sensitivity. Three major "domains" of symptoms associated with schizophrenia are positive or psychotic symptoms, negative/deficit symptoms, and cognitive impairment (Carpenter and Buchanan 1994). Positive or psychotic symptoms, including hallucinations and delusions, are among the most common problems in schizophrenia and are present in 50%–90% of patients (Cutting 1995). Negative symptoms encompass avolition, apathy, anhedonia, asociality, affective flattening, and alogia (Andreasen et al. 1995). The deficit syndrome, negative symptoms due to the disease process of schizophrenia, is present in approximately 25% of patients (Carpenter et al. 1988; Fenton and McGlashan 1994). Neurocognitive impairment is present in 40%–60% of patients with schizophrenia and includes abnormalities in memory, attention, and "executive" or frontal lobe functioning (Goldberg and Gold 1995). Each of these domains of symptoms can interfere with medical care.

Patients with schizophrenia have impaired insight into their psychiatric illness (Amador et al. 1994; McEvoy et al. 1993). Lack of insight appears to be heterogeneous, arising from both neuropsychological deficits and psychological defenses (Amador and Strauss 1993). Many patients with schizophrenia who are unaware of their mental illness are also unaware of comorbid chronic medical illness (J. P. McEvoy, personal communication, January 1996). Noncompliance with psychiatric treatment is also common among people with schizophrenia (Weiden et al. 1995). Although it has not been studied systematically, it is likely that rates of noncompliance with medical treatment among patients with schizophrenia are also high.

Reports dating back to Kraepelin have documented patients with schizophrenia who tolerate pain with little or no discomfort (for review, see Dworkin 1994). For example, Marchand et al. (1959) found that 21% of patients with schizophrenia with acute perforated peptic ulcer and 37% of those with acute appendicitis presented without a complaint of pain. In contrast, pain was a primary complaint in 95% of these cases in the general population. Many case reports provide examples of patients with schizophrenia having severe injuries or suffering from medical conditions without complaints of pain. These include reports of diminished pain in necrotic bowel (Bickerstaff et al. 1988; Rosenthal et al. 1990), fractures (Fishbain 1982; Marchand et al. 1959), myocardial infarctions (Marchand 1955 ; Talbott and Linn 1978), metastatic cancer (Bickerstaff et al. 1988; Talbott and Linn 1978), and severe self-mutilation (Feldman 1988; Talbott and Linn 1978). Diminished pain may lead to delayed or missed diagnoses of concurrent medical illness.

Studies have shown elevated thresholds in patients with schizophrenia for reporting both thermal (Dworkin et al. 1993; Kane et al. 1971) and electrical pain (Buchsbaum et al. 1986; Davis et al. 1979; but see Guieu et al. 1994). A number of hypotheses have been proposed to explain the relative reduction in pain expressed by patients with schizophrenia. Various sociological and psychological factors were outlined by Talbott and Linn (1978). For example, by denying pain, patients can avoid having to adopt the characteristic "sick role" that is usually accompanied by attention from others, nurturance, and cooperation with medical treatment. Research into biological mechanisms have found elevated endorphin levels in patients with schizophrenia (Lindstrom et al. 1986; but see Watson et al. 1979). Altered N-methyl-D-aspartate receptor–mediated neurotransmission (Javitt and Zukin 1991) and antipsychotics (Maltbie et al. 1979) may contribute to reduced pain sensitivity as well. Besides pain insensitivity, patients with schizophrenia also may have proprioceptive defects that could interfere with the ability to monitor and respond to the cues of physical illness (Talbott and Linn 1978). Although such sensory dysfunction has been hypothesized, the experimental evidence remains inconclusive (Leventhal et al. 1982).

Impact of Medical Illness on the Symptoms of Schizophrenia

While schizophrenia can increase the risk of having some medical illness, the impact of medical illness on schizophrenia is less well defined. Historically, many psychiatrists have noted the salutary effect that a serious medical illness can have on psychosis (Clow and Prout 1946; Hinsie 1929; Lipper and Werman 1977; Mayer-Gross et al. 1969; Talbott and Linn 1978). Earlier this century, medical illnesses, including aseptic meningitis and malaria, were actually induced in patients with schizophrenia in an attempt to improve their psychiatric symptoms (Carroll et al. 1925; Warmer 1928). The results were mixed, but a number of these patients experienced such improvement. Other studies found either no consistent correlations between concurrent medical illness and symptoms (Sabbath and Luce 1952; Swartz and Semrad 1951) or an exacerbation of psychotic symptoms (Paneth 1959). Lipper and Werman (1977) noted that none of these studies were prospective, that most lacked controls, and that the criteria for diagnosis were rarely established. Well-controlled investigations remain to be performed.

The role of medical illness has also been addressed in studies of stress and the symptoms of schizophrenia. As reviewed by Norman and Malla (1993), 12 of 14 independent sample groups showed significant correlation between higher levels of stress and worsening of psychotic symptoms among patients with schizophrenia. The stressful events, which were broadly defined but included medical illness, were found to cluster particularly in the 3 weeks prior to the initial onset or exacerbation of psychotic symptoms (Norman and Malla 1993).

Other factors related to physical disease may improve psychotic symptoms. Lipper and Werman (1977) suggested that the increased attention paid to a medically ill patient, and the notion that physical illness may disrupt "habitual" psychotic symptoms, may account for improved psychiatric symptoms in some patients with schizophrenia. Only 51% of patients with schizophrenia and other chronic psychotic illnesses admitted to medical and surgical services required a psychiatric consultation, and the intervention did not reflect acute worsening of psychosis in at least a third of the patients who received a consultation (Gilmore et al. 1994). The majority of patients with schizophrenia appeared to tolerate an acute medical/surgical hospitalization without significant deterioration in symptoms.

Recognition and Management of Medical Illness in Patients With Schizophrenia

Psychiatrists, nonpsychiatrist physicians, and other mental health care providers must be aware of the high prevalence of medical illness in patients with schizophrenia. They also should be alert to the possibility of symptoms that these patients may be unable or unwilling to report. Psychiatrists need to be thorough and persistent in their evaluations of potential medical problems, capable of recognizing and avoiding countertransference and attitudinal factors that limit care for persons with severe mental illness. Koranyi (1979) argued that, because psychiatrists accept unscreened patients, they must screen for medical illnesses through thorough histories, physical exams, and appropriate laboratory tests. Farmer (1987) found that 88% of severely mentally ill persons who attended an intensive community support program could not identify a primary care physician who attended to their outpatient physical health needs. Two-thirds of this sample had their last physical exam on admission to a psychiatric unit.

Several experts have argued that psychiatrists must assume many of the roles of primary care physicians in order to ensure adequate medical care for persons with severe mental illness (Barnes et al. 1983; Koranyi 1979; Oken and Fink 1976). These roles include routine medical screening, other preventive efforts, and care coordination. Patients should be educated so they can make informed choices about their health (Molnar and Fava 1987). It is important to highlight the high rates of smoking and of substance abuse in people with schizophrenia (Drake and Wallach 1989; Goff et al. 1992). Healthy lifestyles, including proper nutrition, physical activity, and "safer sex," should be promoted as much as possible.

The patient's ability to understand and participate in treatment should be assessed. Positive and negative symptoms, neurocognitive dysfunction, and lack of insight can interfere with treatment, and strategies to deal with potential problems should be developed in advance. Steps that may improve treatment compliance include using a straightforward approach with the patient, developing a good relationship with all health care providers, working with the patient's family, and using social services as appropriate (Dickson and Neill 1987). Adler and Griffith (1991) suggest that hospitalized patients with schizophrenia be provided an environment in which procedures and treatments are explained and understood in advance, the routine is predictable, and care providers are consistent. Coordination of care between psychiatrists and other physicians is critical (Adler and Griffith 1991).

Solutions to systemic problems that limit adequate medical care require meaningful health care reform. Expanded eligibility for Medicaid is one way health care reform may benefit people with schizophrenia. As managed care expands its market share in the private sector, Medicaid payments are more appealing to providers, even as states convert Medicaid programs into managed systems of care. Managed-care Medicaid programs are following a variety of models that are expected to have different impacts on general health care (Stroup and Dorwart 1997). In "integrated" managed care programs that require primary care providers to coordinate all care, Medicaid recipients may have improved access to general health care services. Unfortunately, the cost for improved medical care may be decreased access to mental health services, because resources may be diverted toward general medical care. The dominant trend, however, is to "carve out" mental health services to behavioral health managed care organizations. Carve-outs have the advantage of ensuring that mental health funds are not reallocated elsewhere but have the disadvantage that primary care providers can be bypassed and the opportunity for better coordination between psychiatric and general medical care is lost (Stroup and Dorwart 1997). In this model, the need for the psychiatrist to assume the role of the primary care provider is great.

Like all patients with medical illness, those with schizophrenia must provide informed consent prior to treatment. *Informed consent* refers to a patient's right to voluntarily make treatment decisions on the basis of adequate information, their doctor's advice, and other desired inputs. To be valid, informed consent must be obtained voluntarily and must be based on adequate information (Bean et al. 1994). The standard for adequate information is that it should be all the information that a "reasonable" person might need to reach a decision. This includes diagnosis, an explanation of the recommended treatment, and the risks and benefits of the recommended treatment, of alternative treatments, and of no treatment (Appelbaum and Gutheil 1991). Finally, informed consent requires that a person be competent to make the treatment decision at hand (Appelbaum and Gutheil 1991; Bean et al. 1994).

Competence is a legal concept. In determining competence, a judge must balance society's interest in preserving individual autonomy and its wish to protect people from their own poor judgment (Appelbaum and Grisso 1988). Unless someone has been declared legally incompetent, their competence is assumed in day-to-day interactions involving recommended widely accepted treatments. But when a patient refuses a recommended treatment, when a procedure has considerable risk, or when the patient's capacity to make an informed decision is in question, an assessment of competence is required. This type of assessment is for *specific competence* and commonly is made outside a courtroom (Appelbaum and Gutheil 1991). In this situation, psychiatrists are often called on to offer their estimation of what a court would find (Appelbaum and Gutheil 1991). The psychiatrist's role is to gather information about a person's capacity to make a specific decision in order to decide if adjudication of incompetence is necessary (Appelbaum and Grisso 1988).

Specific competence hinges upon a person's capacity to make an autonomous and rational decision about a treatment option and is assessed by four criteria (Appelbaum and Grisso 1988; Appelbaum and Gutheil 1991; Bean et al. 1994). First, a person must be able to communicate his or her wishes. Second, a person must understand information relevant to the treatment decision. Third, the relevant information must be manipulated rationally so that major factors in the decision are "recognizable reasons." Finally, a person must be able to understand their situation and its consequences. The last two criteria leave much discretion to clinicians and potentially allow a great deal of physician discretion and possibly coercion. Commonly, the evaluator employs a "sliding scale" approach to competency that uses different thresholds according to the risk-benefit ratio of a recommended treatment and the evaluator's perception of a rational decision (Appelbaum and Gutheil 1991; Groves and Vaccarino 1987).

Symptoms associated with schizophrenia can interfere with informed consent, both during an acute psychotic episode and during a chronic or residual illness. Although acute psychosis is a common reason for involuntary hospitalization, commitment to a hospital does not imply incompetence to make treatment decisions. Competence must be determined in a separate, formal legal preceding, which would result in the designation of a substitute decision-maker. Jones (1995) argues that cognitive deficits are central to schizophrenia and may persist even with treatment. Since informed consent requires working memory and probabilistic judgment, meaningful informed consent may be illusory even when positive symptoms are absent. Jones noted that neuropsychological tests that model informed consent processes may be helpful in deciding on a patient's ability to give informed consent. Bean et al. (1994) developed an assessment tool—the Competency Interview Schedule—in an attempt to operationalize the concepts of competency for psychiatric patients. Such approaches may help in standardizing assessments and protecting the rights of people with schizophrenia.

Irwin et al. (1985) pointed out that a "consenting" patient who is psychotic may have little actual comprehension of the decision he or she is being asked to make. They suggest that even when a patient with schizophrenia consents to treatment, supplementation by "proxy consent" from a family member may be a rational adjunct. Dickson and Neill (1987) suggested that accepting treatment refusals in nonurgent situations is a helpful approach that may avoid confrontation while leaving open the possibility of later treatment. Such an approach may cause less damage to a therapeutic alliance and is true to the principles of informed consent.

Case Vignette

A 20-year-old homeless man presented to the emergency room with complaints of chest pain and difficulty breathing. Chest X ray revealed significant left pneumothorax. Chest-tube placement and admission were recommended, but the patient, after listening to an explanation of the risks and benefits of the procedure, refused and stated his intention to leave the hospital. Although somewhat irritable, he was cooperative with staff.

The emergency room physician, concerned about the decision to leave the hospital against medical advice, consulted Psychiatry to assess the patient's competence. The patient clearly expressed his desire to leave the hospital. He listened to an explanation of the risks and benefits of a chest tube and the risk of leaving the hospital and was able to repeat the explanations without difficulty. He began to get agitated when questioned about who he would be with, where he would stay, and how he would follow up. He then revealed a psychotic explanation of the origin of his chest pain and the intentions of the emergency room nursing staff. He became extremely agitated and required 4-point restraints.

The psychiatric consultants documented that their evaluation revealed that the patient did not have the capacity to make an informed decision about his medical condition. Surgery was consulted and recommended immediate chest-tube placement as an emergency procedure. The patient was sedated and the chest tube was placed. The patient was discharged from surgery several days later after resolution of his pneumothorax and refusal of voluntary psychiatric hospitalization. He was found not to meet commitment criteria after several days of treatment with neuroleptics.

Summary

Medical illness is common in patients with schizophrenia. Furthermore, patients with schizophrenia are at higher risk for morbidity and mortality associated with some medical illnesses. Schizophrenia, with its associated positive and negative symptoms, neurocognitive abnormalities, and diminished pain sensitivity, can interfere with a patient's ability to recognize symptoms of medical illness, report them to care providers, and engage in treatment. In turn, medical illness can worsen symptoms associated with schizophrenia. All of these factors make the management of medical illness in patients with schizophrenia a complex task.

Psychiatrists should be vigilant to the possibility of medical illness or pregnancy in their patients with schizophrenia. Once a medical illness is recognized, persistence in pursuing an appropriate workup or referral to a primary care care provider is necessary. It is also important to anticipate how symptoms of schizophrenia in an individual patient might interfere with treatment and take steps to minimize their impact on a patient's ability to engage in treatment. In a similar way, the stress associated with medical illness needs to be anticipated and minimized. Finally, psychiatrists need to participate in the assessment of a patient's ability to provide informed consent.

Given the direction in which mental and medical health care systems are evolving under managed care systems, psychiatrists involved in the care of patients with chronic and severe psychiatric illnesses such as schizophrenia will need to accept more responsibility for primary medical care. This responsibility goes beyond recognition and management of medical illness and pregnancy. It includes routine medical screening and education about healthy lifestyles. Psychiatrists who work with the chronic mentally ill have a rich tradition of "psychoeducation"—long an important part of the therapeutic relationship between patient and psychiatrist. Psychoeducation can easily be expanded to include education about issues related to physical health. As awareness of this need to provide aspects of primary medical care grows, the well-documented problems associated with medical illness in patients with schizophrenia can be dealt with more effectively.

References

Adler LE, Griffith JM: Concurrent medical illness in the schizophrenic patient. Epidemiology, diagnosis, and management. Schizophr Res 4:91–107, 1991

Allebeck P: Schizophrenia: a life shortening disease. Schizophr Bull 15:81–89, 1989

Allebeck P, Wistedt B: Mortality in schizophrenia. Arch Gen Psychiatry 43:650–653, 1986

Allebeck P, Rodvall Y, Wistedt B: Incidence of rheumatoid arthritis among patients with schizophrenia, affective psychosis and neurosis. Acta Psychiatr Scand 71:615–619, 1985

Amador XF, Strauss DH: Poor insight in schizophrenia. Psychiatr Q 64:305–318, 1993

Amador XF, Flaum M, Andreasen NC, et al: Awareness of illness in schizophrenia and schizoaffective and mood disorders. Arch Gen Psychiatry 51:826–836, 1994

Andreasen NC, Roy MA, Flaum M: Positive and negative symptoms, in Schizophrenia. Edited by Hirsch SR, Weinberger DR. Cambridge, MA, Blackwell Science, 1995, pp 28–45

Appelbaum PS, Grisso T: Assessing patients' capacities to consent to treatment. N Engl J Med 319:1635–1638, 1988

Appelbaum PS, Gutheil TG: Clinical Handbook of Psychiatry and the Law. Baltimore, MD, Williams & Wilkins, 1991

Baldwin JA: Schizophrenia and physical disease. Psychol Med 9:611–618, 1979

Baldwin JA: Schizophrenia and physical disease: a preliminary analysis of the data from the Oxford Record Linkage Study, in The Biochemistry of Schizophrenia and Addiction. Edited by Hemmings G. Lancaster, UK, MTP Press, 1980, pp 297–318

Barnes RF, Mason JC, Greer C, et al: Medical illness in chronic psychiatric outpatients. Gen Hosp Psychiatry 5:191–195, 1983

Bean G, Nishisato S, Rector NA, et al: The psychometric properties of the Competency Interview Schedule. Can J Psychiatry 39:368–376, 1994

Bickerstaff LK, Harris SC, Leggett RS, et al: Pain insensitivity in schizophrenic patients. A surgical dilemma. Arch Surg 123:49–51, 1988

Black DW: Mortality in schizophrenia—the Iowa Record-Linkage Study: a comparison with general population mortality. Psychosomatics 29:55–60, 1988

Black DW, Warrack G, Winokur G: The Iowa Record-Linkage Study, I: suicides and accidental deaths among psychiatric patients. Arch Gen Psychiatry 42:71–88, 1985

Brugmans J, Verbruggen F, Dom J, et al: Prolactin, phenothiazines, admission to mental hospital, and carcinoma of the breast. Lancet 2:502–503, 1973

Buchsbaum MS, Awsare SV, Holcomb HH, et al: Topographic differences between normals and schizophrenics: the N120 evoked potential component. Biol Psychiatry 15:1–6, 1986

Carpenter WT Jr, Buchanan RW: Schizophrenia. N Engl J Med 330:681–690, 1994

Carpenter WT Jr, Heinrichs DW, Wagman AMI: Deficit and nondeficit forms of schizophrenia: the concept. Am J Psychiatry 145:578–583, 1988

Carroll RS, Barr ES, Barry RG, et al: Aseptic meningitis in the treatment of dementia praecox. Am J Psychiatry 81:673–703, 1925

Clow HE, Prout CT: A study of the modification of mental illness by intercurrent physical disorders in one hundred patients. Am J Psychiatry 103:179–184, 1946

Cournos F, Guido JR, Coomaraswamy S, et al: Sexual activity and risk of HIV infection among patients with schizophrenia. Am J Psychiatry 151:228–232, 1994

Craig TJ, Lin SP: Cancer and mental illness. Compr Psychiatry 22:404–410, 1981

Cutting J: Descriptive psychopathology, in Schizophrenia. Edited by Hirsch SR, Weinberger DR. Cambridge, MA, Blackwell Science, 1995, pp 15–27

Dain N: Reflections on antipsychiatry and stigma in the history of American psychiatry. Hospital and Community Psychiatry 45:1010–1014, 1994

Davis GC, Buchsbaum MS, van Kammen DP, et al: Analgesia to pain stimuli in schizophrenics and its reversal by naltrexone. Psychiatry Res 1:61–69, 1979

D'Ercole A, Skodol AE, Struening E, et al: Diagnosis of physical illness in psychiatric patients using Axis III and a standardized medical history. Hospital and Community Psychiatry 42:395–400, 1991

Dickson LR, Neill JR: When schizophrenia complicates medical care. Am Fam Pract 35:153–159, 1987

Dorian B, Garfinkel PE: Stress, immunity and illness—a review. Psychol Med 17:393–407, 1987

Drake RE, Wallach MA: Substance abuse among the chronic mentally ill. Hospital and Community Psychiatry 40:1041–1046, 1989

Driscoll JS, Melnick NR, Quinn FR, et al: Psychotropic drugs as potential antitumor agents: a selective screening study. Cancer Treatment Reports 62:45–65, 1978

Dworkin RH: Pain insensitivity in schizophrenia: a neglected phenomenon and some implications. Schizophr Bull 20:235–248, 1994

Dworkin RH, Clark WC, Lipsitz JD, et al: Affective deficits and pain insensitivity in schizophrenia. Motivation and Emotion 17:245–276, 1993

Eastwood MR, Stiasny S, Meier R, et al: Mental illness and mortality. Compr Psychiatry 23:377–385, 1982

Ehrentheil OF: Common medical disorders rarely found in psychotic patients. Arch Neurol Psychiatry 77:178–186, 1957

Ettigi P, Lal S, Friessen HG: Prolactin, phenothiazines, admission to mental hospital and carcinoma of the breast. Lancet 2:266–267, 1973

Farmer S: Medical problems of chronic patients in a community support program. Hospital and Community Psychiatry 38:745–749, 1987

Feldman MD: The challenge of self-mutilation: a review. Compr Psychiatry 29:252–269, 1988

Fenton WS, McGlashan TH: Antecedents, symptom progression, and long-term outcome of the deficit syndrome in schizophrenia. Am J Psychiatry 151:351–356, 1994

Fishbain DA: Pain insensitivity in psychosis. Ann Emerg Med 11:630–632, 1982

Gilmore JH, Perkins DO, Lindsey BA: Factors related to psychiatric consultation for schizophrenic patients receiving medical care. Hospital and Community Psychiatry 45:1233–1235, 1994

Goff DC, Henderson, DC, Amico E: Cigarette smoking in schizophrenia: relationship to psychopathology and medication side effects. Am J Psychiatry 149:1189–1194, 1992

Goffman E: Stigma: Notes on the Management of Spoiled Identity. New York, Simon & Schuster, 1963, pp 3–5

Goldberg TE, Gold JM: Neurocognitive deficits in schizophrenia, in Schizophrenia. Edited by Hirsch SR, Weinberger DR. Cambridge, MA, Blackwell Science, 1995, pp 146–162

Gosling RH: Peptic ulcer and mental disorder—II. J Psychosom Res 2:285–301, 1958

Gregg D: The paucity of arthritis among psychotic cases. Am J Psychiatry 95:853–858, 1939

Groves JE, Vaccarino JM: Legal aspects of consultation, in Massachusetts General Hospital Handbook of General Hospital Psychiatry, 2nd Edition. Edited by Hackett TP, Cassem NH. Littleton, MA, PSG Publishing, 1987, pp 591–604

Guieu R, Samuelian JC, Coulouvrat H: Objective evaluation of pain perception in patients with schizophrenia. Br J Psychiatry 164:253–255, 1994

Harris AE: Physical disease and schizophrenia. Schizophr Bull 14:85–96, 1988

Hayward C: Psychiatric illness and cardiovascular disease risk. Epidemiol Rev 17:129–138, 1995

Herrman HE, Baldwin JA, Christie D: A record-linkage study of mortality and general hospital discharge in patients diagnosed as schizophrenic. Psychol Med 13:581–593, 1983

Hinsie LE: The treatment of schizophrenia. Psychiatr Q 3:6–39, 1929

Hussar AE: Peptic ulcer in long-term institutionalized schizophrenic patients. Psychosom Med 30:374–377, 1968

Irwin M, Lovitz A, Marder SR, et al: Psychotic patients' understanding of informed consent. Am J Psychiatry 142:1351–1354, 1985

Javitt DC, Zukin SR: Recent advances in the phencyclidine model of schizophrenia. Am J Psychiatry 148:1301–1308, 1991

Jeste DV, Gladsjo JA, Lindamer LA, et al: Medical comorbidity in schizophrenia. Schizophr Bull 22:413–430, 1996

Jones GH: Informed consent in chronic schizophrenia? Br J Psychiatry 167:565–568, 1995

Kane EM, Nutter RW, Weckowicz TE: Response to cutaneous pain in mental hospital patients. J Abnorm Psychol 1:52–60, 1971

Karasu TB, Waltzman SA, Lindenmayer JP, et al: The medical care of patients with psychiatric illness. Hospital and Community Psychiatry 31:463–472, 1980

Koran LM, Sox HC, Marton KI, et al: Medical evaluation of psychiatric patients. Arch Gen Psychiatry 46:733–740, 1989

Koranyi EK: Morbidity and rate of undiagnosed physical illnesses in a psychiatric clinic population. Arch Gen Psychiatry 36:414–419, 1979

Leventhal DB, Schuck JR, Clemons JT, et al: Proprioception in schizophrenia. J Nerv Ment Dis 170:21–26, 1982

Lieberman AA, Coburn AF: The health of the chronically mentally ill: a review of the literature. Community Ment Health J 22:104–116, 1986

Lindstrom LH, Besev G, Gunne LM, et al: CSF levels of receptor-active endorphins in schizophrenic patients: correlations with symptomatology and monoamine metabolites. Psychiatry Res 19:93–100, 1986

Lipper S, Werman DS: Schizophrenia and intercurrent physical illness: a critical review of the literature. Compr Psychiatry 18:11–22, 1977

Maltbie AA, Cavenar JO, Sullivan JL, et al: Analgesia and haloperidol: a hypothesis. J Clin Psychiatry 40:323–326, 1979

Marchand WE: Occurrence of painless myocardial infarction in psychotic patients. N Engl J Med 253:51–55, 1955

Marchand WE, Sarota B, Marble HC, et al: Occurrence of painless acute surgical disorders in psychotic patients. N Engl J Med 260:580–585, 1959

Masterson E, O'Shea B: Smoking and malignancy in schizophrenia. Br J Psychiatry 145:429–432, 1984

Matthysse S, Lipinski J: Biochemical aspects of schizophrenia. Annu Rev Med 26:551–565, 1975

Mayer-Gross W, Slater E, Roth M: Clinical Psychiatry, 3rd Edition. Baltimore, MD, Williams & Wilkins, 1969, pp 237–262

McCarrick AK, Manderscheid RW, Bertolucci DE, et al: Chronic medical problems in the chronic mentally ill. Hospital and Community Psychiatry 37:289–291, 1986

McEvoy JP, Freter S, Merritt M, et al: Insight about psychosis among outpatients with schizophrenia. Hospital and Community Psychiatry 44:883–884, 1993

Molnar G, Fava GA: Intercurrent medical illness in the schizophrenic patient, in Principles of Medical Psychiatry. Edited by Stoudemire A, Fogel BS. New York, Grune & Stratton, 1987, pp 451–461

Mortensen PB: The occurrence of cancer in first admitted schizophrenic patients. Schizophr Res 12:185–194, 1994

Mortensen PB, Juel K: Mortality and causes of death in first admitted schizophrenic patients. Br J Psychiatry 163:183–189, 1993

Norman RMG, Malla AK: Stressful life events and schizophrenia. Br J Psychiatry 162:161–174, 1993

Oken D, Fink PJ: General psychiatry. A primary-care specialty. JAMA 235:1973–1974, 1976

Paneth HG: Some observations on the relation of psychotic states to psychosomatic disorders. Psychosom Med 21:106–109, 1959

Pilkington TL: The coincidence of rheumatoid arthritis and schizophrenia. J Nerv Ment Dis 124:604–606, 1955

Rosenthal SH, Porter KA, Coffey B: Pain insensitivity in schizophrenia. Case report and review of the literature. Gen Hosp Psychiatry 12:319–322, 1990

Sabbath JC, Luce RA: Psychosis and bronchial asthma. Psychiatr Q 26:562–576, 1952

Simpson JC: Mortality studies in schizophrenia, in Handbook of Schizophrenia, Vol 3: Nosology, Epidemiology and Genetics. Edited by Tsaung MT, Simpson JC. New York, Elsevier, 1988, pp 245–273

Simpson JC, Tsuang MT: Mortality among patients with schizophrenia. Schizophr Bull 22:485–499, 1996

Soni SD, Gill J: Malignancies in schizophrenic patients. Br J Psychiatry 134:447–448, 1979

Sox HC, Koran LM, Sox CH, et al: A medical algorithm for detecting physical disease in psychiatric patients. Hospital and Community Psychiatry 40:1270–1276, 1989

Stefan MD, Catalan J: Psychiatric patients and HIV infection: a new population at risk? Br J Psychiatry 167:721–727, 1995

Stroup TS, Dorwart RA: Overview of public sector managed mental health care, in Managed Mental Health Care in the Public Sector: A Survivors Manual. Edited by Minkoff K, Pollock D. Amsterdam, Gordon & Breech, 1997, pp 1–12

Swartz J, Semrad EV: Psychosomatic disorders in psychoses. Psychosom Med 13:314–321, 1951

Talbott JA, Linn L: Reactions of schizophrenics to life-threatening disease. Psychiatr Q 50:218–227, 1978

Tsuang MT: Suicide in schizophrenics, manics, depressives, and surgical controls. Arch Gen Psychiatry 35:153–155, 1978

Tsuang MT, Woolson RF: Mortality in patients with schizophrenia, mania, depression, and surgical conditions. Br J Psychiatry 130:162–166, 1977

Tsuang MT, Woolson RF: Excess mortality in schizophrenia and affective disorders. Arch Gen Psychiatry 35:1181–1185, 1978

Tsuang MT, Woolson RF, Fleming JA: Premature deaths in schizophrenia and affective disorders: an analysis of survival curves and variables affecting the shortened survival. Arch Gen Psychiatry 37:979-983, 1980

Tsuang MT, Perkins K, Simpson JC: Physical diseases in schizophrenia and affective disorder. J Clin Psychiatry 44:42–46, 1983

Vieweg A, Pandurangi A, Levenson J, et al: Medical disorders in the schizophrenia patient. Int J Psychiatry Med 25:137–172, 1995

Vinogradov S, Gottesman II, Moises HW, et al: Negative association between schizophrenia and rheumatoid arthritis. Schizophr Bull 17:669–678, 1991

Warmer GL: Malarial inoculation in cases of dementia praecox. Psychiatr Q 2:494–505, 1928

Watson SJ, Akil H, Berger PA, et al: Some observations on the opiate peptides and schizophrenia. Arch Gen Psychiatry 36:35–41, 1979

Weiden PJ, Mott T, Curcio N: Recognition and management of neuroleptic noncompliance, in Contemporary Issues in the Treatment of Schizophrenia. Edited by Shriqui CL, Nasrallah HA. Washington, DC, American Psychiatric Press, 1995, pp 411–434

CHAPTER 6

Pregnancy in Patients With Schizophrenia

John H. Gilmore, M.D.
L. Fredrik Jarskog, M.D.
T. Scott Stroup, M.D., M.P.H.

*P*regnancy, while not a medical illness, is usually managed in a medical setting and offers many of the same challenges a medical illness does to the woman with schizophrenia and to physicians providing care. These include recognition of pregnancy and its progression, access to appropriate prenatal care, and the effect of pregnancy on the symptoms and course of schizophrenia. An additional consideration is the pharmacological management of symptoms in the face of potential adverse effects on the fetus. Beyond the pharmacological considerations, women with schizophrenia have high rates of adverse pregnancy outcomes for a variety of reasons.

In this chapter, we offer a review of family planning and pregnancy in patients with schizophrenia. We also review the difficulties associated with the recognition and management of pregnancy in this unique patient population. Suggestions for meeting the challenges that family planning and pregnancy bring to the care of patients with schizophrenia are offered.

Fertility and Family Planning

Fertility rates in women with schizophrenia are lower (30%–80%) compared with the rates among women with other kinds of psychiatric illness and with those in the general population (Haverkamp et al. 1982; Nanko and Moridaira 1993; Saugstad 1989). In addition, reproductive rates decline significantly after the onset of schizophrenia (Saugstad 1989). However,

fertility rates of women with schizophrenia may be increasing (Erlenmeyer-Kimling et al. 1969), and a more recent study found no decrease in
fertility (Burr et al. 1979). This increase in fertility may be related to deinstitutionalization. The recent introduction of newer antipsychotics that
do not elevate prolactin levels also may be increasing fertility rates (Currier and Simpson 1998). For example, there is a recent case report of a
woman who became pregnant after switching to clozapine (Dickson and
Hogg 1998).

Despite potentially reduced fertility rates, women with schizophrenia
do become pregnant. It has been hypothesized that pregnancy in women
with chronic mental illness reflects, in part, a desire for normalcy (Apfel
and Handel 1993). The lack of adequate family planning for women with
schizophrenia and other chronic mental illness is well recognized (Abernethy and Grunebaum 1972; Coverdale et al. 1992, 1993; McCullough et al.
1992; L. J. Miller 1997). Women with schizophrenia and other chronic mental illness are sexually active, lack knowledge about contraception, and
often engage in unprotected sex (Abernethy 1974; Coverdale and Aruffo
1989; Grunebaum et al. 1971; McEvoy et al. 1983). Further, unwanted pregnancies and induced abortions are frequent in this population (Abernethy
1974; Coverdale and Aruffo 1989; Grunebaum et al. 1971; L. J. Miller and
Finnerty 1996; W. H. Miller et al. 1990; Rudolph et al. 1990). Pregnancy for
many women with schizophrenia is characterized by a lack of interpersonal
support and generally poor socioeconomic circumstances (Krener et al.
1989; McNeil et al. 1983; Mowbray et al. 1995). Women with schizophrenia
are more likely to be single mothers (Kumar et al. 1995; McNeil and Kaij
1974; McNeil et al. 1983; Mowbray et al. 1995) or separated from their child
after birth (Coverdale and Aruffo 1989; L. J. Miller and Finnerty 1996;
Mowbray et al. 1995; Rudolph et al. 1990).

Clinical Course of Schizophrenia During Pregnancy

The effect of pregnancy on symptom severity and the course of schizophrenia has not been well studied, but the available data indicate that
pregnancy is often associated with worsening of symptoms. In one study,
9 of 99 women with "endogenous psychoses" had a documented "mental
disturbance" during pregnancy or labor (McNeil and Kaij 1973). In a series
of papers describing pregnancy in 88 women with nonorganic psychosis,
McNeil et al. (1983) found that these women had more nervousness and
anxiety, as well as increased rates of "mental disturbance," during pregnancy than control subjects (McNeil et al. 1984a). More importantly, these
investigators found that 59% of women with schizophrenia experienced

a worsening of mental health during the pregnancy (McNeil et al. 1984b), but only 42% were receiving psychiatric treatment (McNeil et al. 1984a).

The impact of childbirth and the early neonatal period on women with schizophrenia has not been well studied. McNeil and Kaij (1973) found that only 2 of 99 women with endogenous psychoses experienced mental disturbance only in the postpartum period. McNeil (1986) found that 24%–36% of women with schizophrenia in their sample developed postpartum psychosis. Inferences about this period can be gained from the literature on mother-baby psychiatric units. Overall, women with schizophrenia account for only 6%–27% of admissions to such units (Meltzer and Kumar 1985; Kumar et al. 1995; Stewart 1989). In one study, 70% of the admissions of women with schizophrenia were for chronic symptoms, whereas only 30% were for new onset or acute relapse (Kumar et al. 1995). In a group of 24 women with schizophrenia admitted to a mother-baby unit, 22 were admitted for nonacute reasons (Davies et al. 1995). The available evidence suggests that the postpartum period represents a period of relatively higher risk for worsening of symptoms, though not as high as for women with affective illness.

Finally, Yarden et al. (1966) studied the impact of childbirth on the 5-year outcome of married women with schizophrenia. Overall, the study provided evidence that pregnancy and childbirth had no long-lasting impact on the course of the illness in women with chronic schizophrenia. Only when the schizophrenia was acute was childbirth associated with an "aggravating effect," probably due to postponement of effective treatment (Yarden et al. 1966).

Perinatal Complications

The prenatal care of women with schizophrenia and other chronic mental illnesses is often inadequate (W. H. Miller et al. 1990, 1992b). Women with schizophrenia have high rates of obstetric complications during pregnancy and delivery (Sacker et al. 1996; Wrede et al. 1980) and poor perinatal outcome, including neonatal death (Bennedsen 1998; Goodman and Emory 1992; W. H. Miller et al. 1992a; Rieder et al. 1975). Other studies have not found this association between schizophrenia and perinatal complications (Cohler et al. 1975; McNeil and Kaij 1974) or have found the effect limited to first pregnancies (Mizrahi et al. 1974).

The reasons for these poor pregnancy outcomes are many. Noncompliance with prenatal care is an important factor and is associated with homelessness, unemployment, unplanned pregnancy, and psychosis (W. H. Miller et al. 1990). Substance abuse is common among mentally ill pregnant women (W. H. Miller et al. 1990; Rudolph et al. 1990). In addition, women with schizophrenia are more likely than control subjects to have been victims of violence during their pregnancy (L. J. Miller and Finnerty 1996). It has been found that 59%–65% of women with mental illness, including schizophrenia, smoke cigarettes (McNeil et al. 1983; Rudolph et al. 1990). Stress is also associated with low birthweight and prematurity (Wadhwa et al. 1993), and it is possible that the stress associated with a chronic psychotic illness contributes to poor pregnancy outcome. Symptoms associated with schizophrenia can interfere with a woman's ability to understand her pregnancy. For example, one case report described a woman with schizophrenia who believed her enlarging abdomen was being filled by a tumor and tried to destroy it by deliberately falling across chairs, hitting her stomach with her fists, and applying heat to her abdomen (Seymour-Shove et al. 1968). In another case, a woman with schizophrenia performed a cesarean section on herself at home; the infant was healthy and survived (Yoldas et al. 1996).

Psychotic denial of pregnancy is not uncommon. L. J. Miller (1990) found that 12 of 26 women admitted to an inpatient program for the care of pregnant mentally ill women over a 1-year period exhibited some degree of psychotic denial. Denial of pregnancy is associated with a variety of potential risks, including lack of prenatal care and precipitous or unassisted delivery (L. J. Miller 1990). Spielvogel and Wile (1992) found that women with schizophrenia who had psychotic denial of or delusions about their pregnancy were less able to detect the onset of labor. L. J. Miller (1990) noted that psychotic denial decreased with antipsychotic medication and supportive psychotherapy and psychosocial interventions. There is an interesting report in which a pregnant woman with schizophrenia who believed that she really had cancer was convinced she was pregnant only when allowed to see the fetus with ultrasound (Cook and Howe 1984).

Management of Pregnancy in Women With Schizophrenia

Family planning should be discussed with all female patients who are of child-bearing potential. Given the potential for denial, clinicians should be alert to the possibility of an unrecognized pregnancy. If a female patient with schizophrenia does become pregnant, it is important to assess her capacity to care for herself, risk factors such as smoking and substance abuse, access to prenatal care, and her ultimate ability to take care of the child. Referral to appropriate prenatal care, social services, and psychiatric treatment should be made. The care of a woman with schizophrenia who is psychotic, in denial about her pregnancy, or engaging in behavior that is potentially dangerous to the fetus brings up many ethical and legal dilemmas related to informed consent (Mahowald and Abernethy 1985; Kolder et al. 1987) and civil commitment in order to protect the fetus (Dal Pozzo and Marsh 1987; Soloff et al. 1979).

The use of psychotropic medication during pregnancy has been extensively reviewed by several authors (Altshuler and Szuba 1994; Altshuler et al. 1996; Cohen et al. 1989; Hauser 1985; Kerns 1986; L. J. Miller 1991, 1994a; Mortola 1989; Nurnberg and Prudic 1984; Robinson et al. 1986; Stowe and Nemeroff 1995). Overall, the use of psychotropic medication during pregnancy requires weighing the risks of potential harm to the fetus against the risk of worsening psychotic symptoms. Withholding psychopharmacotherapy during pregnancy involves the "general" risks of disruption of functioning, prolonged hospitalization, vulnerability to suicide or violence, and potential loss of jobs, housing, or social support. It also involves risks related to pregnancy: malnutrition, attempts at premature self-delivery, fetal abuse or neonaticide, refusal of prenatal care, and precipitous delivery (L. J. Miller 1991). Altshuler et al. (1996) consider acute psychosis during pregnancy a medical and obstetrical emergency.

All routinely used psychotropic medications, including antipsychotics, lithium, antidepressants, benzodiazepines, and anticonvulsants, cross the placenta (Mortola 1989; Nurnberg and Prudic 1984). The risks of using psychotropic medication during pregnancy encompass five broad categories: teratogenic effects, effects on labor and delivery, toxic effects on the fetus and neonate, long-term behavioral effects, and effects on the breast-feeding infant (Robinson et al. 1986). Although an initial study of phenothiazines found a higher-than-expected incidence of congenital malformations in children exposed to chlorpromazine in utero (Rumeau-Rouquette et al. 1977), other studies found no such increase (Milkovich and Van den Berg 1976; Slone et al. 1977; but see Edlund and Craig 1984). Other studies have found no increase in fetal abnormalities in women taking other classes of antipsychotics (Kerns 1986; Mortola 1989; Robinson et al. 1986). Robinson et al. (1986) concluded that "despite many years of widespread use of neuroleptics, there have been relatively few reports of malformations" (p. 184).

A variety of symptoms have been noted in the newborn exposed to antipsychotic medication in utero, including extrapyramidal symptoms, jaundice, respiratory depression, functional bowel obstruction, and behavioral abnormalities (L. J. Miller 1991). Studies of children exposed in utero to antipsychotics have not revealed any significant long-lasting effects on IQ or behavior (L. J. Miller 1991; Robinson et al. 1986). Little is known about the risks of the agents used to treat extrapyramidal side effects, though diphenhydramine, benztropine, and trihexyphenidyl have been associated with minor malformations (L. J. Miller 1994a), and their use should be avoided. Beta-blockers have not been associated with congenital abnormalities and can be used to treat akathisia during pregnancy (L. J. Miller 1994a).

Other psychotropic medications are often used as adjuvant treatment in women with schizophrenia, and their use will be briefly discussed. Lithium has been associated with Ebstein's anomaly of the heart, and though the risk is probably much lower than previously thought, its use should be avoided during pregnancy when possible, especially in the first trimester (Cohen et al. 1994). Carbamazepine and valproate are associated with neural tube defects and likewise should be avoided when possible, especially in the first trimester (Stowe and Nemeroff 1995). Diazepam has been associated with oral clefts, though the findings from studies are contradictory; other benzodiazepines have not been associated with congenital anomalies (L. J. Miller 1991, 1994a). Tricyclic antidepressants have not been associated with congenital malformations in large, systematic studies (Altshuler and Szuba 1994; L. J. Miller 1994a). There are few data on monoamine oxidase inhibitors, serotonin reuptake inhibitors, and other newer antidepressants (Stowe and Nemeroff 1995). Finally, electroconvulsive therapy has been used safely during pregnancy (L. J. Miller 1994b; Walker and Swartz 1994) and may be considered.

Most authors recommend avoiding antipsychotics during the first trimester if possible (Altshuler and Szuba 1994; Cohen et al. 1989; Hauser 1985; L. J. Miller 1991; Mortola 1989; Robinson et al. 1986; Stowe and Nemeroff 1995). Informed consent should be obtained prior to beginning or continuing medication during pregnancy. When antipsychotics are used during pregnancy, high-potency drugs are recommended, because chlorpromazine has a possible risk of congenital abnormalities and low-potency drugs with significant hypotensive effects may cause uteroplacental insufficiency (Hauser 1985; Mortola 1989). Cohen et al. (1989) pointed out that maintenance low-dose antipsychotics may prevent the need for higher doses during an acute psychotic episode and, perhaps, higher risk of adverse effects on the fetus. If possible, medication might be reduced or stopped 5–10 days prior to the expected delivery date to minimize effects on the neonate (L. J. Miller 1991).

If a woman with schizophrenia wants to get pregnant, the decision to discontinue medication should be carefully considered. The small but potential risks to the fetus must be weighed against the likelihood of relapse and the severity of relapse in the individual patient. Guidelines for targeted-intermittent medication approaches in nonpregnant patients with schizophrenia may aid the decision-making process. General contraindications to targeted use of antipsychotics include significant baseline symptoms that would interfere with the ability to function, current stress, history of uncooperativeness with treatment, and a history of suicidal or violent behavior (Chiles et al. 1989). The presence of a medical condition that might worsen in the face of psychotic relapse is also considered a contraindication to intermittent medication (Chiles et al. 1989); pregnancy might be considered a medical condition in this sense. Robinson et al. (1986) recommended that conception be attempted only after a period of relative stability, that periods of known stress or risk of relapse be avoided, and that medication be stopped several weeks prior to anticipated conception. The periods of maximum risk for teratogenicity—4–10 weeks after fertilization—should be as medication free as possible (L. J. Miller 1991). A strategy for the treatment of a relapse, should it occur during pregnancy, should be planned with the patient in advance (Cohen et al. 1989).

Case Vignette

A 40-year-old woman with a diagnosis of schizoaffective disorder was admitted to the OB-GYN service for abnormal bleeding and was found to be several weeks' pregnant. A danger of spontaneous abortion passed, and the patient indicated that she wanted to continue the pregnancy. Psychiatry was consulted to help manage the patient because she appeared to be mildly psychotic. She had been compliant with her medications (lithium, carbamazepine, and haloperidol), and her doctors requested a recommendation regarding continuation of the medications.

History taking revealed that during a previous pregnancy the patient's medications were discontinued and she suffered a severe decompensation that necessitated long-term hospitalization. From this information and a careful review of the evidence of the teratogenicity of lithium and carbamazepine, the psychiatric consultants recommended continuation of all her medications. The patient was alert and oriented despite mild psychotic symptoms, and responded appropriately to explanations of the risks and benefits of continuing to take lithium and the other psychotropic medication. She was reminded of her previous experience off medications and readily agreed with the doctors' recommendation. The consultants documented that the patient's reason for continuing her medication was based on a rational manipulation of the information presented and was not due to a psychotic process that did not hold up to the "recognizable reason" standard.

Summary

Pregnancy offers many of the same challenges as medical illness does to patients with schizophrenia and their physicians. Patients with schizophrenia are at high risk for complications and adverse outcomes during pregnancy. Schizophrenia, with its associated positive and negative symptoms, neurocognitive abnormalities, and diminished pain sensitivity, can interfere with a patient's ability to recognize pregnancy and complications of pregnancy, report them to care providers, and engage in treatment. Pregnancy can worsen symptoms associated with schizophrenia. All these factors make the management of pregnancy in patients with schizophrenia a complex task.

Psychiatrists should discuss family planning with their patients with schizophrenia and be attentive to the possibility of pregnancy. Once pregnancy is recognized, proper referral to a prenatal care provider is necessary. The risks and benefits of continuing medication during pregnancy need to be assessed and discussed. It is important to anticipate how symptoms of schizophrenia in an individual patient might interfere with prenatal care as well as the care of the infant after birth. With a heightened awareness of how the illness of schizophrenia can impact the course of pregnancy, many of the problems associated with pregnancy in patients with schizophrenia can be minimized.

References

Abernethy V: Sexual knowledge, attitudes, and practices of young female psychiatric patients. Arch Gen Psychiatry 30:180–182, 1974

Abernethy VD, Grunebaum H: Toward a family planning program in psychiatric hospitals. Am J Public Health 62:1638–1646, 1972

Altshuler LL, Szuba MP: Course of psychiatric disorders in pregnancy. Dilemmas in pharmacologic management. Neurol Clin 12:613–635, 1994

Altshuler LL, Cohen L, Szuba MP, et al: Pharmacologic management of psychiatric illness during pregnancy: dilemmas and guidelines. Am J Psychiatry 153:592–606, 1996

Apfel RJ, Handel MH: Madness and Loss of Motherhood: Sexuality, Reproduction, and Long-Term Mental Illness. Washington, DC, American Psychiatric Press, 1993

Bennedsen BE: Adverse pregnancy outcome in schizophrenia women: occurrence and risk factors. Schizophr Res 33:1–26, 1998

Burr WA, Falek A, Strauss LT, et al: Fertility in psychiatric outpatients. Hospital and Community Psychiatry 30:527–531, 1979

Chiles JA, Sterchi D, Hyde T, et al: Intermittent medication for schizophrenic outpatients: who is eligible? Schizophr Bull 15:117–121, 1989

Cohen LS, Heller VL, Rosenbaum JF: Treatment guidelines for psychotropic drug use in pregnancy. Psychosomatics 30:25–33, 1989

Cohen LS, Friedman JM, Jefferson JW, et al: A reevaluation of risk of in utero exposure to lithium. JAMA 271:146–150, 1994

Cohler BJ, Gallant DH, Grunebaum HU, et al: Pregnancy and birth complications among mentally ill and well mothers and their children. Soc Biol 22:269–278, 1975

Cook PE, Howe B: Unusual use of ultrasound in a paranoid patient (letter). Can Med Assoc J 131:539, 1984

Coverdale JH, Aruffo JA: Family planning needs of female chronic psychiatric outpatients. Am J Psychiatry 146:1489–1491, 1989

Coverdale J, Aruffo J, Grunebaum H: Developing family planning services for female chronic mentally ill outpatients. Hospital and Community Psychiatry 43: 475–478, 1992

Coverdale JH, Bayer TL, McCullough LB, et al: Respecting the autonomy of chronic mentally ill women in decisions about contraception. Hospital and Community Psychiatry 44:671–674, 1993

Currier GW, Simpson GM: Antipsychotic medications and fertility. Psychiatr Serv 49:175–176, 1998

Dal Pozzo EE, Marsh FH: Psychosis and pregnancy: some new ethical and legal dilemmas for the physician. Am J Obstet Gynecol 156:425–427, 1987

Davies A, McIvor RJ, Kumar RC: Impact of childbirth on a series of schizophrenic mothers: a comment on the possible influence of oestrogen on schizophrenia. Schizophr Res 16:25–31, 1995

Dickson RA, Hogg L: Pregnancy of a patient treated with clozapine. Psychiatr Serv 49:1081–1083, 1998

Edlund MJ, Craig TJ: Antipsychotic drug use and birth defects: an epidemiologic reassessment. Compr Psychiatry 25:32–37, 1984

Erlenmeyer-Kimling L, Nicol S, Rainer JD, et al: Changes in fertility rates of schizophrenic patients in New York State. Am J Psychiatry 125:916–927, 1969

Goodman SH, Emory EK: Perinatal complications in births to low socioeconomic status schizophrenic and depressed women. J Abnorm Psychol 101:225–229, 1992

Grunebaum HU, Abernethy VD, Rofman ES, et al: The family planning attitudes, practices, and motivations of mental patients. Am J Psychiatry 128:740–744, 1971

Hauser LA: Pregnancy and psychiatric drugs. Hospital and Community Psychiatry 36:817–818, 1985

Haverkamp F, Propping P, Hilger T: Is there an increase of reproductive rates in schizophrenics? I. Critical review of the literature. Archiv für Psychiatrie und Nervenkrankheiten 232:439–450, 1982

Kerns LL: Treatment of mental disorders in pregnancy: a review of psychotropic drug risks and benefits. J Nerv Ment Dis 174:652–659, 1986

Kolder VEB, Gallagher J, Parsons MT: Court-ordered obstetrical interventions. N Engl J Med 316:1192–1196, 1987

Krener P, Simmons MK, Hansen RL, et al: Effect of pregnancy on psychosis: life circumstances and psychiatric symptoms. Int J Psychiatry Med 19:65–84, 1989

Kumar R, Marks M, Platz C, et al: Clinical survey of a psychiatric mother and baby unit: characteristics of 100 consecutive admissions. J Affect Disord 33:11–22, 1995

Mahowald M, Abernethy V: When a mentally ill woman refuses abortion. Hastings Cent Rep 15:22–23, 1985

McCullough LB, Coverdale J, Bayer T, et al: Ethically justified guidelines for family planning interventions to prevent pregnancy in female patients with chronic mental illness. Am J Obstet Gynecol 167:19–25, 1992

McEvoy JP, Hatcher A, Appelbaum PS, et al: Chronic schizophrenic women's attitudes toward sex, pregnancy, birth control and childrearing. Hospital and Community Psychiatry 34:536–539, 1983

McNeil TF: A prospective study of postpartum psychoses in a high-risk group. 1. Clinical characteristics of the current postpartum episodes. Acta Psychiatr Scand 74:205–216, 1986

McNeil TF, Kaij L: Obstetric notations of mental or behavioral disturbance. J Psychosom Res 17:175–188, 1973

McNeil TF, Kaij L: Reproduction among female mental patients: obstetric complications and physical size of offspring. Acta Psychiatr Scand 50:3–15, 1974

McNeil TF, Kaij L, Malmquist-Larsson A: Pregnant women with nonorganic psychosis: life situation and experience of pregnancy. Acta Psychiatr Scand 68:445–457, 1983

McNeil TF, Kaij L, Malmquist-Larsson A: Women with nonorganic psychosis: mental disturbance during pregnancy. Acta Psychiatr Scand 70:127–139, 1984a

McNeil TF, Kaij L, Malmquist-Larsson A: Women with nonorganic psychosis: pregnancy's effect on mental health during pregnancy. Acta Psychiatr Scand 70:140–148, 1984b

Meltzer ES, Kumar R: Puerperal mental illness, clinical features and classification: a study of 142 mother-and-baby admissions. Br J Psychiatry 147:647–654, 1985

Milkovich L, Van den Berg BJ: An evaluation of the teratogenicity of certain antinauseant drugs. Am J Obstet Gynecol 125:244–248, 1976

Miller LJ: Psychotic denial of pregnancy: phenomenology and clinical management. Hospital and Community Psychiatry 41:1233–1237, 1990

Miller LJ: Clinical strategies for the use of psychotropic drugs during pregnancy. Psychiatr Med 9:275–298, 1991

Miller LJ: Psychiatric medication during pregnancy: understanding and minimizing risks. Psychiatric Annals 24:69–75, 1994a

Miller LJ: Use of electroconvulsive therapy during pregnancy. Hospital and Community Psychiatry 45:444–450, 1994b

Miller LJ: Sexuality, reproduction, and family planning in women with schizophrenia. Schizophr Bull 23:623–635, 1997

Miller LJ, Finnerty M: Sexuality, pregnancy, and childrearing among women with schizophrenia-spectrum disorders. Psychiatr Serv 47:502–506, 1996

Miller WH, Resnick MP, Williams MH, et al: The pregnant psychiatric inpatient: a missed opportunity. Gen Hosp Psychiatry 12:373–378, 1990

Miller WH, Bloom JD, Resnick MP: Chronic mental illness and perinatal outcome. Gen Hosp Psychiatry 14:171–176, 1992a

Miller WH Jr, Bloom JD, Resnick MP: Prenatal care for pregnant chronic mentally ill patients. Hospital and Community Psychiatry 43:942–943, 1992b

Mizrahi MirDal GK, Mednick SA, Schulsinger F, et al: Perinatal complications in children of schizophrenic mothers. Acta Psychiatr Scand 50:553–568, 1974

Mortola JF: The use of psychotropic agents in pregnancy and lactation. Psychiatr Clin North Am 12:69–87, 1989

Mowbray CT, Oyserman D, Zemencuk JK, et al: Motherhood for women with serious mental illness: pregnancy, childbirth, and the postpartum period. Am J Orthopsychiatry 65:21–38, 1995

Nanko S, Moridaira NS: Reproductive rates in schizophrenic outpatients. Acta Psychiatr Scand 87:400–404, 1993

Nurnberg HG, Prudic J: Guidelines for treatment of psychosis during pregnancy. Hospital and Community Psychiatry 35:67–71, 1984

Rieder RO, Rosenthal D, Wender P, et al: The offspring of schizophrenics: fetal and neonatal deaths. Arch Gen Psychiatry 32:200–211, 1975

Robinson GE, Stewart DE, Flak E: The rational use of psychotropic drugs in pregnancy and postpartum. Can J Psychiatry 31:183–190, 1986

Rudolph B, Larson GL, Sweeny S, et al: Hospitalized pregnant psychotic women: characteristics and treatment issues. Hospital and Community Psychiatry 41:159–163, 1990

Rumeau-Rouquette C, Goujard J, Huel G: Possible teratogenic effect of phenothiazines in human beings. Teratology 15:57–64, 1977

Sacker A, Done DJ, Crow TJ: Obstetric complications in children born to parents with schizophrenia: a meta-analysis of case-control studies. Psychol Med 26:279–287, 1996

Saugstad LF: Social class, marriage, and fertility in schizophrenia. Schizophr Bull 15:9–43, 1989

Seymour-Shove R, Gee DJ, Cross AP: Schizophrenia during pregnancy associated with injury to foetus in utero. BMJ 1(593):686, 1968

Slone D, Siskind V, Heinonen OP, et al: Antenatal exposure to the phenothiazines in relation to congenital malformations, perinatal mortality rate, birth weight, and intelligence quotient score. Am J Obstet Gynecol 128:486–488, 1977

Soloff PH, Jewell S, Roth LH: Civil commitment and the rights of the unborn. Am J Psychiatry 136:114–115, 1979

Spielvogel A, Wile J: Treatment and outcomes of psychotic patients during pregnancy and childbirth. Birth 19:131–137, 1992

Stewart DE: Psychiatric admission of mentally ill mothers with their infants. Can J Psychiatry 34:34–38, 1989

Stowe ZN, Nemeroff CB: Psychopharmacology during pregnancy and lactation, in The American Psychiatric Press Textbook of Psychopharmacology. Edited by Schatzberg AF, Nemeroff CB. Washington, DC, American Psychiatric Press, 1995, pp 823–837

Wadhwa PD, Sandman CA, Porto M, et al: The association between prenatal stress and infant birth weight and gestational age at birth: a prospective investigation. Am J Obstet Gynecol 169:858–865, 1993

Walker R, Swartz CM: Electroconvulsive therapy during high-risk pregnancy. Gen Hosp Psychiatry 16:348–353, 1994

Wrede G, Mednick SA, Huttunen MO, et al: Pregnancy and delivery complications in the births of an unselected series of Finnish children with schizophrenic mothers. Acta Psychiatr Scand 62:369–381, 1980

Yarden PE, Max DM, Eisenbach Z: The effect of childbirth on the prognosis of married schizophrenic women. Br J Psychiatry 112:491–499, 1966

Yoldas Z, Iscan A, Yoldas T, et al: A woman who did her own caesarean section (letter). Lancet 348:135, 1996

CHAPTER 7

Cognitive Impairment in Older Schizophrenia Patients

J. Akiko Gladsjo, Ph.D.
John H. Eastham, Pharm.D.
Dilip V. Jeste, M.D.

With increases in life expectancy and changes in the demographic composition of the United States population, the prevalence of dementia and the number of older schizophrenia patients are expected to increase considerably. Thus, there is a growing need for specialized management and treatment options tailored to the needs of the older patient. Most treatment protocols, however, were developed for younger adults and may be unsuitable for older patients, who may have comorbid medical conditions or increased sensitivity to medication side effects.

Some of the confusion surrounding the diagnosis of dementia is related to the evolving meaning of the term itself. Kraepelin used the term *dementia praecox* ("precocious dementia") to refer to the psychotic disorder with a deteriorating course of personality functioning, especially in terms of volition and other cognitive abilities now thought to be subserved by the frontal lobes (Kraepelin 1919/1971). Although Kraepelin described loss of intellect and knowledge as a key feature of this disorder, the term *dementia* did not have the same connotation as it does today. E. Bleuler

This work was supported, in part, by National Institute for Mental Health grants MH49671, MH45131, and MH43693 and by the Department of Veterans Affairs.

(cited by Karno and Norquist 1989) used a broader definition of the illness that included conditions of patients who did not demonstrate a deteriorating course. He acknowledged that schizophrenia was accompanied by a loss of various cognitive abilities but believed that this deterioration tended to occur in the earlier stages of the disorder, leaving memory and comprehension largely intact. His son, M. Bleuler (1968), noted that severe cognitive impairment was a relatively rare occurrence: only 5%–15% of schizophrenia patients had acute deterioration, while an additional 10%–20% displayed "chronic deterioration."

Other research addressing the prevalence of dementia in late-life schizophrenia has yielded conflicting results. Some longitudinal and cross-sectional studies that investigated cognitive decline in schizophrenia suggest that schizophrenia is associated with a stable cognitive deficit rather than a progressive dementia (Goldberg et al. 1993b; Heaton et al. 1994). Ciompi (1980), in a 37-year longitudinal follow-up of a large sample of schizophrenia patients, found that 58% of the sample presented with no manifestations or very minor manifestations of "psycho-organic" deterioration, whereas only 8% presented with severe dementia. He concluded that significant cognitive deterioration was relatively rare in schizophrenia.

Although frank dementia may be considered uncommon in schizophrenia, it remains an important concern because of the burden it adds to the care of the patient with schizophrenia. Cost of care is one practical issue that must be taken into account when treating older schizophrenia patients. Schizophrenia is one of the most expensive mental disorders in terms of treatment costs, loss of productivity, and public assistance payments (Rice and Miller 1996; Wyatt et al. 1995). The total cost of schizophrenia in the United States is estimated to be about $33 billion annually. A recent study examining patterns and costs of mental health service use in the United States (Cuffel et al. 1996) found that total direct and indirect costs for schizophrenia were higher than those for any other psychiatric disorder. The increased costs were not distributed evenly over the schizophrenia patient population. Instead, the youngest and oldest patients accounted for significantly higher average annual expenditures compared with individuals in the 30- to 65-year age range. This pattern of costs stands in contrast to that seen in service use and costs for other psychiatric disorders, which generally decrease with age. Although Cuffel et al.'s study did not investigate the specific causes for the increased treatment expense, it was noted that late-onset schizophrenia, increased medical comorbidity, sequelae of substance abuse, and cognitive impairment all may contribute to higher care costs for older schizophrenia patients. Even when older persons are free from mental illness or cognitive impairment, they account for a larger proportion of health care costs than their younger counterparts because of physical comorbidity (National Institute on Aging 1987).

In this chapter, we discuss definitions, diagnostic criteria, epidemiology, patient assessment, differential diagnosis, and management of cognitive impairment (including dementia) in older patients with schizophrenia.

Definitions and Diagnostic Criteria

The diagnostic category of dementia in DSM and other diagnostic systems has evolved as more research on the pathophysiology of cognitive impairment has accumulated. Initially, the hallmark of dementia was thought to be an irreversible course. As new treatments were developed, it became clear that some dementias (e.g., those due to hypothyroidism, normal-pressure hydrocephalus) were reversible with appropriate treatment. Next, progressive deterioration was identified as the characteristic feature of dementia. Eventually, however, the diagnostic category was broadened to include static encephalopathies, such as those due to head injury and cerebral vascular accidents. The most recent DSM dementia criteria require only deterioration from a previous level of cognitive functioning (American Psychiatric Association 1994), but there is no requirement of the time course over which this must occur, and there is no connotation regarding future deterioration.

The essential feature of DSM-IV diagnosis of dementia is the development of multiple cognitive deficits, with the cardinal symptom of memory impairment and at least one other cognitive deficit (Table 7–1). Other criteria include impairment in occupational or social functioning and evidence of a decline from a higher level of functioning. In DSM-IV, almost all the dementia diagnoses are specific to particular etiologies (e.g., vascular dementia). Some categories (e.g., dementia of the Alzheimer's type) specifically require that the disturbance not be better accounted for by another Axis I disorder, such as schizophrenia, which decreases the likelihood that these disorders would be diagnosed concurrently.

As previously noted, the diagnosis of dementia in patients with schizophrenia is controversial for several reasons.

Overlap in Diagnostic Criteria

Both schizophrenia and dementia require impairment in social or occupational functioning. Since the majority of individuals with schizophrenia

Table 7–1. DSM-IV-TR diagnostic criteria for dementia (Criteria A, B, and D/E only)

A. The development of multiple cognitive deficits manifested by both
   (1) memory impairment (impaired ability to learn new information or to recall previously learned information)
   (2) one (or more) of the following cognitive disturbances:
      (a) aphasia (language disturbance)
      (b) apraxia (impaired ability to carry out motor activities despite intact motor function)
      (c) agnosia (failure to recognize or identify objects despite intact sensory function)
      (d) disturbance in executive functioning (i.e., planning, organizing, sequencing, abstracting)
B. The cognitive deficits in Criteria A1 and A2 each cause significant impairment in social or occupational functioning and represent a significant decline from a previous level of functioning.
D./E. The deficits do not occur exclusively during the course of a delirium.

Source. Adapted with permission from American Psychiatric Association: *Diagnostic and Statistical Manual of Mental Disorders*, 4th Edition, Text Revision. Washington, DC, American Psychiatric Association, 2000. Copyright 2000, American Psychiatric Association.

have neuropsychological deficits, it can be difficult to determine the etiology of cognitive impairment presenting in an elderly patient. It is often unclear whether poor performance on cognitive tests and impaired daily functioning are due to schizophrenia alone, an independent dementia, or some interaction of these two processes. Cohen et al. (1988) found that elderly schizophrenia patients residing in the community peformed significantly worse on the Dementia Rating Scale (Mattis 1973), with scores below the cutoff for dementia, than did demographically matched control subjects. It has also been suggested that schizophrenia patients' poor cognitive performance may be related to the interference by psychotic symptoms, medication effects, poor motivation, and deleterious effects of chronic hospitalization.

Another difficulty arises in diagnosing dementia in patients with schizophrenia, because many individuals with schizophrenia may have technically met the criteria for dementia (i.e., cognitive deterioration) at or shortly after their first break. One study, which compared executive functioning in younger schizophrenia inpatients (average age = 33 years) with elderly individuals without schizophrenia residing in nursing homes or residential care (average age = 86 years), found no differences in performance between the two groups, despite differences in age and neuroleptic use (Royall et al. 1993). Elderly schizophrenia patients are likely to have cognitive impairment secondary to aging as well as to schizophrenia. One way to clarify whether the cognitive impairment with which schizophrenia patients present is related to psychosis or dementia is to examine patients' neuropsychological profiles before and after the alleged development of dementia. This type of information is rarely available, however, especially for very chronic, elderly patients.

Variability in the Definition of Memory

A number of studies examining neuropsychological functioning in patients with schizophrenia have reported impaired memory (e.g., McKenna et al. 1990; Saykin et al. 1994), some in the context of a generalized cognitive deficit and others with the suggestion of a selective deficit in memory. There is a lack of consensus, however, regarding exactly how memory should be operationalized. Patients (or caregivers) may report subjective problems with memory when the actual deficit is in attention, learning, or recall. Some studies assert the presence of memory impairment when subjects have poor recall of a prose passage (e.g., Saykin et al. 1994) or a geometric figure. For example, McKenna et al. (1990) reported the existence of a selective amnestic disorder in approximately 50% of a sample of schizophrenia patients who ranged in age from 18 to 68 years and were recruited from a broad range of treatment facilities. The observed memory deficit was considered to be disproportionately greater than the schizophrenia patients' overall intellectual impairment. However, the authors' conclusion was based on a limited battery of tests and the use of a test that did not dissociate the separate processes of learning, recall, and recognition memory. Thus, their finding of a "selective amnesia" might have been an artifact of the test employed.

Other researchers have attempted to parse memory functioning into separate learning, recall, and recognition memory functions. Discrepancies in the neuropsychological research findings can be explained by variability in terminology and assessment methods. For example, Heaton et al. (1994) noted the importance of distinguishing between efficiency with which new information is learned and the ability to recall information after a delay. Studies using the California Verbal Learning Test (Delis et al. 1987), a word-list learning task that separately evaluates learning, free and cued short-term and long-term recall, and recognition memory, have found that schizophrenia patients have impaired learning but relatively intact recognition memory (Paulsen et al. 1995). Gold et al. (1992) also reported that when initial level of learning was controlled for, schizophrenia patients had a normal rate of forgetting, although learning was impaired. Until there is some agreement on the type of "memory loss" required for the diagnosis of dementia, this will remain a controversial area.

Epidemiology

The frequency of dementia in individuals with schizophrenia is not known. Reported prevalence varies widely with the diagnostic criteria and assessment methods used and the setting (outpatient vs. institution) in which the data are gathered. There are numerous methodological impediments to understanding the prevalence and severity of dementia, including the confounding of psychiatric symptoms and cognitive impairment, subject dropout, and the impact of comorbid medical conditions. As discussed earlier, a lack of concensus on the definition of comorbid dementia in schizophrenia contributes to confusion about prevalence. Consequently, it may be more appropriate to ask how common cognitive impairment (rather than dementia) in schizophrenia is. Despite methodological divergence across studies, it appears that at least three-fourths of the patients with schizophrenia have some degree of significant cognitive impairment (Palmer et al. 1996; Silverstein and Zerwic 1985). The overall pattern of cognitive deficits in schizophrenia may not be related to age at onset or duration of illness (Heaton et al. 1994; Hyde et al. 1994; Jeste et al. 1995) but instead represents a core feature of schizophrenia secondary to underlying brain pathology.

Cross-Sectional Studies

Several groups of researchers have inferred an absence of significant cognitive deterioration over time from cross-sectional studies involving patients with varying duration of illness. One cross-sectional study (Hyde et al. 1994) that addressed the issue of cognitive decline in schizophrenia found no differences among five age cohorts ranging from 18 to 69 years of age on tests sensitive to dementia, including the Mini-Mental State Exam (MMSE; Folstein et al. 1975). The authors inferred that, although schizophrenia patients' cognitive functioning was significantly impaired compared with healthy individuals, their neuropsychological functioning did not decline significantly over the course of their disorder. In their review of more than 100 studies that focused on the effects of aging in schizophrenia, Heaton and Drexler (1987) concluded that the cognitive deficits associated with schizophrenia were not strongly affected by aging, although the literature was marked by many methodological limitations. With the exception of a small subset of patients, cognitive performance in most schizophrenia patients appeared to be relatively stable and was not associated with progressive deterioration despite chronic illness or long-term institutionalization. Instead, the apparent dementia observed in the older schizophrenia patients may have been secondary to depression, medication side effects, alcohol and drug use, or comorbid medical problems.

Setting

One reason for a lack of consistent findings on cognitive impairment in schizophrenia is that few studies have included truly representative samples drawn from large populations of older schizophrenia patients in the community. Most studies draw subjects from a single sample of convenience, such as a single clinic or inpatient ward, and their results reflect the characteristics of that target population. Thus, studies of long-term inpatient populations report relatively high prevalence of dementia and severe cognitive impairment, whereas research with stable outpatients has found relatively low rates of dementia (e.g., Heaton et al. 1994). It appears that the select groups of patients left in institutions and skilled nursing facilities are those who are most impaired in their ability to function independently and have been least amenable to rehabilitation (Soni and Mallik 1993). For instance, Johnstone et al. (1981) followed 120 patients for approximately 7 years after an acute psychotic episode and found significant differences in cognitive functioning between patients who were currently hospitalized and those who were residing in the community at follow-up. Current inpatients performed worse on all measures of cognitive ability, although the two groups did not differ in terms of negative or positive psychotic symptoms.

Some evidence supporting the notion of a relative rarity of Alzheimer's-type dementia in patients with schizophrenia comes from the work of Paulsen et al. (1995), who examined the learning and memory profiles of schizophrenia outpatients. These investigators found that only 15% of the patients had learning and memory performances consistent with a cortical dementia pattern. In contrast, some researchers studying populations of institutionalized elderly schizophrenia patients have reported high rates of dementia. For example, Davidson and Haroutunian (1995) reported that 60% of chronically institutionalized schizophrenia patients had dementia, with MMSE scores near zero. Despite the severity of impairment, the authors asserted that the cognitive profile of deficits could be distinguished from that seen in Alzheimer's disease patients. A 2-year follow-up of these patients (Harvey et al. 1995) found little change in their cognitive functioning, providing evidence for the notion that cognitive impairment in geriatric schizophrenia, though sometimes severe, is not due to Alzheimer's disease. It is possible that the detection of cognitive deterioration was limited by "floor effects," in that most patients scored near zero at the first assessment, leaving little room to observe deterioration. Several other research groups (Arnold et al. 1995b; Kincaid et al. 1995) studying chronically institutionalized, elderly schizophrenia patients have reported high rates of severe dementia, ranging from 36% to 100%.

Variability in the Diagnostic Criteria for Schizophrenia and Dementia

Many of the older studies did not use formal diagnostic criteria or assessment methods, relying only on clinical judgment, whereas more recent studies have used a variety of diagnostic systems: Research Diagnostic Criteria (RDC; Feighner et al. 1972), DSM-III (American Psychiatric Association 1980), or DSM-III-R (American Psychiatric Association 1987). It has been noted that different definitions and diagnostic criteria of schizophrenia have different prognostic implications (Kendell et al. 1981; Stephens et al. 1980), particularly for symptom outcome. When diagnostic criteria require the presence of deterioration in functioning, it is not surprising that outcomes are skewed toward impaired functioning and chronicity (Carpenter and Strauss 1991). In contrast, when diagnostic criteria rely on cross-sectional positive symptoms, such as the RDC for schizophrenia, outcomes are more heterogeneous. Angst's (1988) review of European studies concluded that diagnostic concepts of schizophrenia were too diverse to allow meaningful conclusions regarding course and outcome.

Some studies required face-to-face, structured clinical interviews for diagnosis, whereas others were based on chart review alone. Several studies (Arnold et al. 1995b; Harvey et al. 1992) examined the concordance of dementia ratings of elderly schizophrenia patients generated from chart review and those derived from patient, caregiver, and chart information. Half of all "chart diagnoses" were inaccurate, compared with diagnoses derived from a comprehensive interview, and dementia severity was systematically overestimated when only chart records were used. Differences in exclusion criteria may also account for some discrepancies in study results. A few studies have used conservative, test performance–based criteria to screen out dementias due to comorbid medical conditions (Cohen et al. 1988; Perlick et al. 1992), whereas other studies are more liberal in their subject inclusion criteria.

Longitudinal Studies

Because reported prevalence of dementia in schizophrenia varies with setting, the best estimates of incidence may come from long-term prospective studies. Unfortunately, most studies of longitudinal outcome in schizophrenia have focused primarily on clinical symptoms and have often neglected the separate assessment of cognitive abilities. Thus, even when studies included as measures of functioning important domains such as work, relationships, self-care, and use of treatment, the investigators generally did not determine whether poor functioning was related to psychopathology, cognitive problems, or both.

Ciompi (1980) conducted one of the largest and best-known longitudinal follow-up studies of dementia in patients with schizophrenia. Beginning with 1,642 cases, he followed 289 surviving patients for an average of 37 years and completed a comprehensive evaluation that included patient and collateral informant interviews and review of all available records. Subjects with schizophrenia had a mortality rate 1.37 times that in the general population, with patients with catatonic-subtype schizophrenia having the highest mortality rate (2.5 times the rate in the general population). Differences in mortality rates were thought to have a net "favorable selection effect" on group outcome. A tendency toward "calming and improving" of symptoms over time was noted, while negative symptoms, such as indifference, abulia, and withdrawal, tended to predominate in old age. Less than 10% of elderly schizophrenia patients developed severe dementia with amnesia and temporal disorientation. Although impressive in terms of length of follow-up, the study had some weaknesses—for example, cognitive functioning was not formally assessed, and severity of psychopathology and cognitive deficits were apparently confounded on at least one of the clinical rating measures.

Neuropathological Studies

Many studies have examined the structural abnormalities present in the brains of schizophrenia patients, but only a few have focused on those with comorbid dementia. Because Alzheimer's disease is the most common cause of dementia in the elderly, most of these studies have looked for Alzheimer's-type pathology in the brains of elderly schizophrenia patients. Although their generalizability may be limited by the selected subgroups studied, these findings may further our understanding of the risk factors and causes of dementia in schizophrenia.

In one postmortem study (Powchik et al. 1993), involving a small sample of chronically institutionalized, geriatric schizophrenia patients, the brains were examined for the neuritic plaques and neurofibrillary tangles characteristic of Alzheimer's disease. Although these patients had been characterized as severely cognitively impaired via retrospective clinical ratings, none of the brains showed evidence of plaques or tangles. Another small neuropathological study, which analyzed the brains of 10 chronically hospitalized elderly patients with both schizophrenia and dementia diagnosed according to DSM-III-R criteria, found that only one patient had brain pathology consistent with Alzheimer's disease (Arnold et al. 1994). Eight of the 10 subjects were considered devoid of pathology that could account for dementia. Several other studies reported that neuropathological characteristics of Alzheimer's disease were "virtually never observed" in patients with schizophrenia and other cognitively impaired patients (Arnold et al. 1995a; Casanova et al. 1993).

Although most studies have reported low rates of Alzheimer's-type pathology, two exceptions have been reported. Prohovnik et al. (1993) studied chronically institutionalized elderly patients and found that 28% of schizophrenia patients had an Alzheimer's-like neuropathology at autopsy. A provocative study by Wisniewski et al. (1994) analyzed the brains of 102 elderly schizophrenia patients for neurofibrillary tangles and neuritic plaques and reported a significant increase in numerical density of neurofibrillary tangles and evidence of accelerated degeneration of neurons in patients who had been treated with neuroleptics. The incidence of neurofibrillary tangles was more than twice as high in the neuroleptic-treated patients (74%) as in those who had died in the preneuroleptic era (36%). These researchers proposed that chronic treatment with neuroleptics, rather than the schizophrenia itself, was associated with earlier and accelerated development of neurofibrillary tangles. This surprising finding needs confirmation. It is possible that methodological differences may explain divergence in the neuropathological studies. Overall, however, it seems that Alzheimer's-type pathology is rare in schizophrenia.

Patient Assessment and Differential Diagnosis

A number of medical conditions can present as dementia (Table 7–2). Because many clinicians expect adaptive-functioning deficits in schizophrenia patients, it is possible to overlook other sources of impaired cognition.

If dementia is observed in an elderly psychotic patient, a comprehensive medical workup is indicated to rule out medication side effects, substance or alcohol abuse, untreated depression, neurological and other physical comorbidity, or sensory impairment as a possible cause of the cognitive impairment. Once other causes have been ruled out, it is useful

---

Table 7–2. Medical conditions that may present as "dementia"

Medication side effects

Major depressive disorder

Substance abuse/dependence

Exposure to toxic agents (e.g., solvents, heavy metals)

Infectious diseases (e.g., neurosyphilis, HIV)

Endocrine disorders

Metabolic disorders

Cardiovascular disorders

Malnutrition

Normal-pressure hydrocephalus

Seizure disorder

Sensory impairments

---

to assess the patient's current level of cognitive status with one of the many brief, standardized instruments available for this purpose. The MMSE (Folstein et al. 1975) and the Dementia Rating Scale (Mattis 1973) are two of the most widely used screening tests that have proved useful in both clinical and research settings. Both tests are brief, easy to administer, and useful for monitoring changes in cognitive functioning. Below we discuss some common causes of severe cognitive impairment in schizophrenia patients.

Medication Side Effects

Adverse effects of drugs, including drug-drug interactions, represent one of the most common, reversible causes of impaired cognitive functioning in the elderly psychiatric patient. As people age, they tend to require lower doses of medications because of changes in metabolism, liver function, or synergistic effects with other medications. In assessing a schizophrenia patient who has had a recent decline in cognitive status, it is important to take a careful and comprehensive medical history to determine whether medication effects account for the changes in cognition. It may be useful to consult with caregivers or with other treating physicians in order to collect accurate, current dosage information. A quick perusal of the *Physicians' Desk Reference* (1996) indicates that many medications are associated with low but significant rates of cognitive side effects. Anticholinergic medications and tricyclic antidepressants are both known to have deleterious effects on cognitive functioning (Spohn and Strauss 1989), especially in older patients. Nonpsychotropic drugs, such as corticosteroids, may also produce impairment of memory and other cognitive abilities. It is also important to evaluate for use or misuse of over-the-counter medications. Antihistamines and over-the-counter cold preparations, in particular, may account for mental dullness, confusion, and other cognitive difficulties that may be misdiagnosed as dementia. Patients may take too much of these medications because of misunderstanding about proper dosing, confusion, memory difficulties, or even delusional ideas.

Age-related memory disturbances are believed to be due to muscarinic dysfunction (Bartus et al. 1982), and medications with anticholinergic (muscarinic-blocking) properties are likely to worsen memory function in the elderly. Anticholinergic medications used in high doses can impair cognitive function, and some, but not all, studies have reported cognitive impairment even with medications used in therapeutic doses (Stern et al. 1987; Thienhaus et al. 1990; Tollefson et al. 1991; Tune and Coyle 1981). In a study of learning and memory, Paulsen et al. (1995) found a modest negative correlation between total learning and daily anticholinergic dose in a large sample of schizophrenia patients. Several nonpsychotropic medications not generally associated with noticeable anticholinergic activity (i.e., cimetidine, digoxin, and furosemide) may have detectable anticholinergic effects and may impair memory and attention in elderly patients (Tune et al. 1992).

Major Depression

Major depression is a frequent cause of memory complaints in elderly individuals. Diminished ability to think or concentrate is one of the nine diagnostic criteria for major depression in DSM-IV and may be perceived by patients as a sign that they are "losing their mind" or becoming demented. This phenomenon has been called "pseudo-dementia," although this term has fallen out of favor (Jeste et al. 1990). Depressive symptoms may affect individuals with schizophrenia, especially those with relatively intact insight and higher intellect. As noted earlier, schizophrenia negatively affects all life domains and patients' coping ability, resulting in depressed mood. As patients age, they may reminisce, evaluate their lives, and compare themselves with their siblings or friends who have lived unaffected by severe mental illness. In elderly patients, memory complaints that are not confirmed by caregiver observations may be explained by comorbid depression. Age-related differences in the patient gender ratio may also account for an increased prevalence of depression in elderly schizophrenia patients. Female schizophrenia patients are more likely to experience affective symptoms (Goldstein and Link 1988; Lewine 1985), and women may be overrepresented in samples of elderly patients. If depression is suspected, the patient should be carefully assessed for other symptoms of mood disturbance, including changes in sleep, appetite, energy level, feelings of hopelessness and worthlessness, and suicidal ideation. In Chapter 2 (this volume), Siris describes a number of possible etiologic factors that should be considered when evaluating a schizophrenic individual with depression. Antidepressant treatment should be pursued if appropriate, because comorbid depression responds about as well as uncomplicated depression. Alternatively, as noted in Chapter 2, a change in neuroleptic medication or treatment philosophy may be helpful for managing comorbid depression.

Comorbid Alcohol or Other Substance Abuse/Dependence

As noted in Chapter 7 (this volume), comorbid alcohol or other substance abuse/dependence represents an important cause of impaired cognitive functioning in individuals with schizophrenia. Data from the Epidemiologic Catchment Area study indicate that substance abuse disorders were the most common comorbid disorders seen in schizophrenia patients. Lifetime prevalence of alcohol abuse or dependence in persons with schizophrenia (meeting DSM-III-R criteria) was 3.3 times higher than that in the general population, with 33% of the schizophrenic individuals affected (Regier et al. 1990).

Although estimates of the prevalence of substance abuse disorders in schizophrenia vary widely because of study differences, it is clear that substance abuse disorders should not be overlooked as a possible cause of cognitive impairment. Chronic substance abuse may cause frank cognitive impairment in individuals who are free from other psychiatric problems (Parsons et al. 1987). More recent research (Duke et al. 1994) that examined alcohol use in patients with schizophrenia demonstrated that higher alcohol use was associated with more severe psychiatric symptoms and more disturbed behaviors that could mimic dementia. In our sample of older schizophrenia patients (mean age = 60 years), the prevalence of DSM-III-R-diagnosed past alcohol abuse or dependence (31%) was almost four times that of comparison subjects (Jeste et al. 1996b). Use of illicit drugs, such as marijuana (Negrete et al. 1986) and cocaine (Brady et al. 1990), has also been shown to be associated with more severe psychiatric symptoms and worse prognosis (see Chapter 9, this volume, for discussion of the effects of specific substances).

Clinicians may find brief screening questionnaires such as the Michigan Alcoholism Screening Test (MAST; Seltzer 1971) and the Drug Abuse Screening Test (Skinner 1982) to be helpful adjuncts for recognizing problem substance use. Although some psychiatrists regularly assess their younger patients for drug and alcohol use, they may neglect to make such an assessment with their elderly patients. It may be especially helpful to administer such tests when evaluating patients with impaired cognitive functioning. Liver function tests, specifically GGTP, and urine toxicology tests may also be helpful in identifying individuals with substance use disorders.

Environmental Exposures to Toxic Chemicals

Environmental exposure to toxic chemicals has also been implicated as a cause of cognitive impairment and even permanent dementia. Individuals may be exposed to solvents and heavy metals such as lead, mercury, and arsenic in the workplace or at home. Symptoms vary depending on the type of chemical exposure. If toxic exposure is suspected, it is important to assess for sources of both acute and long-term exposure. Although removal of the offending agent may improve symptoms, some individuals may be left with a residual persisting condition.

Medical Disorders

A number of physical illnesses may result in mental status changes (Jeste et al. 1996b). Patients with chronic schizophrenia often experience barriers to adequate diagnosis and treatment of these comorbid disorders, such as lack of insurance and trouble communicating their needs clearly to their physicians. Although some of the physical illnesses may be reversed with proper treatment, others may cause permanent dementia and disabilities. For example, untreated HIV infection and neurosyphilis may cause progressive dementia with significant impact on functional abilities.

Anemia, vitamin B_{12} and folate deficiencies, hypothyroidism, and other medical conditions may affect cognitive functioning. Poor nutrition secondary to impaired ability to carry out activities of daily living may result in a vicious cycle leading to impaired cognition. Elderly individuals also may be at a particularly high risk for electrolyte imbalances. For example, diuretic medications prescribed for hypertension may cause hypokalemia. Some schizophrenia patients, especially long-term institutionalized patients, may develop hyponatremia secondary to polydipsia (deLeon et al. 1992; Jos et al. 1986).

Some schizophrenia patients may develop chronic obstructive pulmonary disease or other cardiovascular diseases secondary to a lifetime of heavy smoking. Chronic hypoxemia secondary to chronic obstructive pulmonary disease may compromise cerebral functioning proportional to hypoxemic severity.

Normal-pressure hydrocephalus is another possible cause of cognitive decline with which the elderly patient may present. Although this condition is relatively rare, it is important to evaluate for this treatable cause of dementia. A comprehensive neurological examination that includes evaluation of the classic triad of "magnetic gait," incontinence, and insidious cognitive decline would be instructive. A head computed tomography scan (or magnetic resonance imaging) and lumbar puncture may be useful for making the diagnosis.

Another low-probability disorder that may be considered is a seizure disorder. Postictal states and absence seizures may be mistaken for dementia. Neuroleptic medications, especially low-potency neuroleptics, are known to lower seizure threshold and may exacerbate a seizure disorder. It is important to take a careful history from the caregiver, as well as the patient, to determine possible causes of seizure onset, such as head injury. An electroencephalogram may be useful for detecting a seizure disorder, although false negative results are more common in elderly patients.

Whereas many of these diagnostic procedures would routinely be considered for the older nonpsychiatric individual, they tend to be neglected for the older schizophrenia patient. Research has shown that patients with schizophrenia receive less and poorer general health care than do their nonpsychiatric peers (Koranyi 1979). For example, Koranyi (1979) examined detection of physical illnesses by physicians who referred patients to a psychiatric clinic and found that nonpsychiatrist physicians missed one-third of their patients' comorbid medical conditions. Another study, which examined prevalence of physical disease in psychiatric patients in the California public health system, reported that only 47% of patients' physical illnesses were recognized by mental health staff (Koran et al. 1989). Among the undiagnosed medical conditions, 16% were considered "causative" (i.e., entirely responsible for the presenting psychiatric symptoms). Some researchers (Talbott and Linn 1978) have noted that older patients with chronic schizophrenia are less likely to verbalize pain or discomfort that would alert clinicians to their health problems.

Sensory Impairment

Hearing impairment is one of the most common medical problems in the geriatric population, with approximately 25% of individuals between the ages of 65 and 74 and 50% of individuals over age 75 affected. Difficulty in understanding speech or misinterpretation of what others are saying due to hearing loss may manifest as a problem in comprehension, attention, or memory. Kreeger et al. (1995), using a crossover design, investigated the impact of hearing deficits on mental status ratings in geriatric psychiatric patients. The researchers found that patients displayed less psychopathology when they were assessed while wearing a functional hearing aid. Elderly schizophrenia patients may be at a particular disadvantage in getting appropriate correction for their hearing deficits (Prager and Jeste 1993). Anecdotally, some physicians have reported trouble assessing sensory functioning in psychotic patients. Nonpsychiatrist doctors may have trouble determining if a patient's complaints of hearing strange noises represent an auditory hallucination or a sign of hearing impairment. Careful screening can help determine whether sensory deficits account for apparent dementia.

Management

Cognitive impairment is a frequent problem associated with schizophrenia that has high costs for both society and the individual in terms of quality of life. Most treatments, however, target only the psychotic symptoms, and these treatments sometimes have adverse effects on cognitive functioning (Cassens et al. 1990; Medalia et al. 1988; Spohn and Strauss 1989). Furthermore, the clinical symptoms of psychosis may wax and wane while the neuropsychological problems associated with schizophrenia persist. We agree with Davidson and Keefe (1995) that cognitive impairment should be considered a target for pharmacological treatment of schizophrenia. Cognitive impairment is clearly important in terms of treatment planning and placement decisions. Ability to carry out activities of daily living, such as self-care, is related to cognitive performance (Heaton and Pendleton 1981; Royall et al. 1993).

In a review of the literature examining the relationship between neurocognitive deficits and daily functioning, Green (1996) found that psychotic symptoms were not significantly related to outcome in any of the studies reviewed. Although the studies varied widely in methodology, cognitive abilities assessed, and patient populations studied, several consistent findings emerged. Verbal memory had the strongest association with all types of functional outcome. Vigilance or attention was associated with social problem solving and skill acquisition; this finding is notable in that both Kraepelin and Bleuler saw attentional problems as a key part of schizophrenia. Performance on the Wisconsin Card Sorting Test (Heaton 1981) was related to community functioning. Negative symptoms predicted difficulties with social problem solving. Green's findings further support the notion that cognitive functioning represents a useful target for treatment.

Dementia in older schizophrenia patients may lead to special management problems that affect treatment compliance, transportation, and activities of daily living. For example, the risk of medication noncompliance would be expected to be greater in individuals with memory and executive function deficits. Problems with attention, learning, and memory may limit the ability to benefit from rehabilitation interventions, social skills training, and even basic psychoeducation. Higher rates of physical comorbidity in older schizophrenia patients may complicate treatment because of the direct and indirect effects of comorbid illnesses and multiple medications. There is growing evidence that elderly nursing home residents with dementia syndromes complicated by other Axis I disorders are considered more uncooperative and receive more staff interventions and use of restraints (Rovner et al. 1992). Other authors have reported that cognitive impairment in patients with schizophrenia contributes to longer acute hospitalizations and earlier admissions to nursing homes (Keefe et al. 1994).

The first step in the management of a schizophrenia patient with dementia (or at least significant cognitive impairment) is assessment for and treatment of any potentially reversible condition listed in the previous section (e.g., major depression). Specific pharmacological management of dementia in patients with schizophrenia is a difficult proposition given the limited treatments that are currently available (Davidson and Keefe 1995). Treatment of behavior problems in patients with other dementias (i.e., primary degenerative or multi-infarct dementia) has generally involved the use of benzodiazepines and neuroleptics. Benzodiazepines are sometimes useful in treating angry outbursts or severe hostility in acute situations, but they do not improve the overall dementia and may in fact impair cognitive functioning. The use of typical neuroleptics for controlling agitation in patients with dementia generally results in modest improvement (Schneider et al. 1990). No single agent among the typical neuroleptics seems to be more efficacious than any other in treating dementia-associated agitation (Lohr et al. 1992). Because neuroleptics are the mainstay of schizophrenia treatment and dementia may develop in patients with schizophrenia, continued use of a typical agent probably has no additional effect on the evolving dementia.

Atypical antipsychotics (serotonin-dopamine D_2 receptor antagonists) are newer agents for treating psychoses. Atypical agents that are currently approved for use in the United States are clozapine, risperidone, olanzapine, and quetiapine. Only a few studies have examined the effects of atypical antipsychotic agents on neuropsychological function.

Studies of clozapine that examined neuropsychological functioning have reported conflicting results. Goldberg et al. (1993a) assessed the effect of clozapine in 15 young patients with treatment-resistant illness (mean age = 35 years), primarily with schizophrenia. Although the patients showed improvement in psychopathology, the treatment did not result in improved performance on neuropsychological assessments. Clozapine use was actually associated with impaired performance on several measures, including tests of problem solving and psychomotor speed. In contrast, Hagger et al. (1993), in a study that examined the cognitive effects of clozapine in 36 young patients with treatment-resistant schizophrenia, found mild but significant improvements on tests of executive function, attention, and memory after 6 months of clozapine treatment. Clozapine treatment was also associated with significant improvements in psychopathology, as measured on the Brief Psychiatric Rating Scale (Overall and Gorham 1962). However, there was no significant relationship between changes in psychopathology and improvement in scores on neuropsychological measures.

Several small studies have indicated that risperidone may enhance global cognition in elderly psychotic patients. In an open-label study (Borison et al. 1994), the cognitive effects of risperidone were assessed in a subset of 22 patients with schizophrenia or Alzheimer's disease (mean age = 69.8 years), who were all experiencing psychotic symptoms at baseline. After 3 weeks of receiving 6 mg/day of risperidone, MMSE and Digit Symbol test scores increased but other cognitive test scores remained essentially unchanged. A second open-label study involved 10 elderly patients with schizophrenia (mean age = 71 years) (Berman et al. 1996). After at least 3 weeks of risperidone treatment, overall psychopathology as measured by the Positive and Negative Syndrome Scale (Kay et al. 1987) decreased significantly, whereas performance on most of the cognitive test scores improved. We assessed the cognitive effects of risperidone in an open-label study (Jeste et al. 1996a) in a group of 19 psychotic patients, most of whom carried a diagnosis of schizophrenia. Patients (mean age = 64.7 years) were administered risperidone for 10.6 ± 7.0 weeks, at doses ranging from 0.5 to 6 mg/day (mean dose = 3 mg/day). Mean MMSE scores increased significantly from baseline scores.

There is a critical need for large-scale, double-blind studies in this area. In the only such double-blind study reported, Berman et al. (1995) compared cognitive effects of risperidone and haloperidol in 20 geriatric patients with schizophrenia but no dementia (mean age = 67.4 years). Both groups showed improvement in positive symptoms, but only the patients in the risperidone group tended to exhibit improvement in negative symptoms. Patients in the risperidone group showed improvements in MMSE scores, whereas patients receiving haloperidol essentially exhibited no significant changes on other cognitive measures.

Summary

There is still much to be learned about comorbid dementia in schizophrenia. The prevalence of dementia in schizophrenia is unknown, but cognitive impairment is very common. Only rigorous, longitudinal, prospective studies will be able to identify the factors that predict the course and outcome of cognitive functioning in patients with schizophrenia, the relationship between psychotic symptoms and cognitive functioning, and the nature of dementia in schizophrenia. Given that the outcome appears to be related in part to cognitive functioning, researchers and clinicians need to reconsider what symptoms represent the most appropriate targets for treatment in the elderly schizophrenia patient.

References

American Psychiatric Association: Diagnostic and Statistical Manual of Mental Disorders, 3rd Edition. Washington, DC, American Psychiatric Press, 1980

American Psychiatric Association: Diagnostic and Statistical Manual of Mental Disorders, 3rd Edition, Revised. Washington, DC, American Psychiatric Press, 1987

American Psychiatric Association: Diagnostic and Statistical Manual of Mental Disorders, 4th Edition. Washington, DC, American Psychiatric Association, 1994

Angst J: European long-term followup studies of schizophrenia. Schizophr Bull 14:501–513, 1988

Arnold SE, Franz BR, Trojanowski JQ: Elderly patients with schizophrenia exhibit infrequent neurodegenerative lesions. Neurobiol Aging 15:299–303, 1994

Arnold SE, Franz BR, Gur RC, et al: Smaller neuron size in schizophrenia in hippocampal subfields that mediate cortical-hippocampal interactions. Am J Psychiatry 152:738–748, 1995a

Arnold SE, Gur RE, Shapiro RM, et al: Prospective clinicopathologic studies of schizophrenia: accrual and assessment of patients. Am J Psychiatry 152:731–737, 1995b

Bartus RT, Dean RL, Beer B, et al: The cholinergic hypothesis of geriatric memory dysfunction. Science 217:408–417, 1982

Berman I, Merson A, Allan E, et al: Effect of risperidone on cognitive performance in elderly schizophrenic patients: a double-blind comparison with haloperidol. Poster presented at the 35th annual meeting of the New Clinical Drug Evaluation Unit, Boca Raton, FL, May 29–June 3, 1995

Berman I, Merson A, Rachov-Pavlov J, et al: Risperidone in elderly schizophrenic patients: an open-label trial. Am J Geriatr Psychiatry 4:173–179, 1996

Bleuler M: A 23-year longitudinal study of 208 schizophrenics and impressions in regard to the nature of schizophrenia, in The Transmission of Schizophrenia. Edited by Rosenthal D, Kety SS. New York, Pergamon, 1968, pp 3–12

Borison RL, Davidson M, Berman I: Risperidone treatment in elderly patients with schizophrenia or dementia. Poster presented at the 46th Institute of Hospital and Community Psychiatry meeting, 1994

Brady KT, Anton RF, Ballenger JC, et al: Cocaine abuse among schizophrenic patients. Am J Psychiatry 147:1164–1167, 1990

Carpenter WT, Strauss JS: The prediction of outcome in schizophrenia IV: eleven year follow-up of the Washington IPSS cohort. J Nerv Ment Dis 179:517–525, 1991

Casanova MF, Carosella NW, Gold JM, et al: A topographical study of senile plaques and neurofibrillary tangles in the hippocampi of patients with Alzheimer's disease and cognitively impaired patients with schizophrenia. Psychiatry Res 49:41–62, 1993

Cassens G, Inglis AK, Appelbaum PS, et al: Neuroleptics: effects on neuropsychological function in chronic schizophrenic patients. Schizophr Bull 16:477–499, 1990

Ciompi L: Catamnestic long-term study on the course of life and aging of schizophrenics. Schizophr Bull 6:606–618, 1980

Cohen CI, Stastny P, Perlick D: Cognitive deficits among aging schizophrenic patients residing in the community. Hospital and Community Psychiatry 39:557–559, 1988

Cuffel BJ, Jeste DV, Halpain M, et al: Treatment costs and use of community mental health services for schizophrenia by age-cohorts. Am J Psychiatry 153:870–876, 1996

Davidson M, Haroutunian V: Cognitive impairment in geriatric schizophrenic patients, in Psychopharmacology: The Fourth Generation of Progress. Edited by Bloom FE, Kupfer DJ. New York, Raven, 1995, pp 1447–1549

Davidson M, Keefe RSE: Cognitive impairment as a target for pharmacological treatment in schizophrenia. Schizophr Res 17:123–129, 1995

deLeon J, Simpson GM, Peralta V: Positive and negative symptoms in schizophrenia: where are the data? Biol Psychiatry 31:431–434, 1992

Delis DC, Kramer JH, Kaplan E, et al: California Verbal Learning Test (CVLT) Manual. New York, Psychological Corporation, 1987

Duke PJ, Pantelis C, Barnes TR: South Westminster Schizophrenia Survey: alcohol use and its relationship to symptoms, tardive dyskinesia and illness onset. Br J Psychiatry 164:630–636, 1994

Feighner JP, Robins E, Guze SB, et al: Diagnostic criteria for use in psychiatric research. Arch Gen Psychiatry 26:57–63, 1972

Folstein MF, Folstein SE, McHugh PR: Mini-Mental State: a practical method for grading the cognitive state of patients for the clinician. J Psychiatr Res 12:189–198, 1975

Gold JM, Randolph C, Carpenter CJ, et al: Forms of memory failure in schizophrenia. J Abnorm Psychol 101:487–494, 1992

Goldberg TE, Greenberg RD, Griffin SJ, et al: The effect of clozapine on cognition and psychiatric symptoms in patients with schizophrenia. Br J Psychiatry 162:43–48, 1993a

Goldberg TE, Hyde TM, Kleinman JE, et al: Course of schizophrenia: neuropsychological evidence for a static encephalopathy. Schizophr Bull 19:797–804, 1993b

Goldstein JM, Link BG: Gender and the expression of schizophrenia. J Psychiatr Res 2:141–155, 1988

Green MF: What are the functional consequences of neurocognitive deficits in schizophrenia? Am J Psychiatry 153:321–330, 1996

Hagger C, Buckley P, Kenny JT, et al: Improvement in cognitive functions and psychiatric symptoms in treatment-refractory schizophrenic patients receiving clozapine. Biol Psychiatry 34:702–712, 1993

Harvey PD, Davidson M, Powchik P, et al: Assessment of dementia in elderly schizophrenics with structured rating scales. Schizophr Res 7:85–90, 1992

Harvey PD, White L, Parrella M, et al: The longitudinal stability of cognitive impairment in schizophrenia. Mini-Mental State scores at one- and two-year follow-ups in geriatric in-patients. Br J Psychiatry 166:630–633, 1995

Heaton RK. A Manual for the Wisconsin Card Sorting Test. Odessa, FL, Psychological Assessment Resources, 1981

Heaton RK, Drexler M: Clinical neuropsychological findings in schizophrenia and aging, in Schizophrenia and Aging. Edited by Miller NE, Cohen GD. New York, Guilford, 1987, pp 145–161

Heaton RK, Pendleton MG: Use of neuropsychological tests to predict adult patients' everyday functioning. J Consult Clin Psychol 49:807–821, 1981

Heaton R, Paulsen J, McAdams LA, et al: Neuropsychological deficits in schizophrenia: relationship to age, chronicity and dementia. Arch Gen Psychiatry 51: 469–476, 1994

Hyde TM, Nawroz S, Goldberg TE, et al: Is there cognitive decline in schizophrenia? A cross-sectional study. Br J Psychiatry 164:494–500, 1994

Jeste DV, Gierz M, Harris MJ: Pseudodementia: myths and reality. Psychiatric Annals 20:71–79, 1990

Jeste DV, Harris MJ, Krull A, et al: Clinical and neuropsychological characteristics of patients with late-onset schizophrenia. Am J Psychiatry 152:722–730, 1995

Jeste DV, Eastham JH, Lacro JP, et al: Management of late-life psychosis. J Clin Psychiatry 57 (suppl 3):39–45, 1996a

Jeste DV, Gladsjo JA, Lindamer LA, et al: Medical comorbidity in schizophrenia. Schizophr Bull 22:413–430, 1996b

Johnstone EC, Owens DGC, Gold A, et al: Institutionalization and the defects of schizophrenia. Br J Psychiatry 139:195–203, 1981

Jos CJ, Evenson RC, Mallya AR: Self-induced water intoxication: a comparison of 34 cases with matched controls. J Clin Psychiatry 47:368–370, 1986

Karno M, Norquist GS: Schizophrenia, in Comprehensive Textbook of Psychiatry/V, 5th Edition, Vol 1. Edited by Kaplan HI, Sadock BJ. Baltimore, MD, Williams & Wilkins, 1989, pp 699–815

Kay SR, Fiszbein A, Opler LA: The Positive and Negative Syndrome Scale (PANSS) for schizophrenia. Schizophr Bull 13:261–276, 1987

Keefe RSE, Blum C, Harvey PD, et al: Working memory deficits in schizophrenia with severe self-care regulation (abstract). Schizophr Res 11:158, 1994

Kendell RE, Brockington IF, Leff JP: Prognostic implications of six alternative definitions of schizophrenia. Arch Gen Psychiatry 36:25–31, 1981

Kincaid MM, Harvey PD, Parrella M, et al: Validity and utility of the ADAS-L for measurement of cognitive and functional impairment in geriatric schizophrenic inpatients. J Neuropsychiatry Clin Neurosci 7:76–81, 1995

Koran LM, Sox HC, Marton KI, et al: Medical evaluation of psychiatric patients. Arch Gen Psychiatry 46:733–740, 1989

Koranyi EK: Morbidity and rate of undiagnosed physical illnesses in a psychiatric clinic population. Arch Gen Psychiatry 36:414–419, 1979

Kraepelin E: Dementia Praecox and Paraphrenia (1919). Translated by Barclay RM. Huntington, NY, Krieger, 1971

Kreeger JL, Raulin ML, Grace J, et al: Effect of hearing enhancement on mental status ratings in geriatric psychiatric patients. Am J Psychiatry 152:629–631, 1995

Lewine R: Schizophrenia: an amotivational syndrome in men. Can J Psychiatry 30:316–318, 1985

Lohr JB, Jeste DV, Harris MJ, et al: Treatment of disordered behavior, in Clinical Geriatric Psychopharmacology. Edited by Salzman C. Baltimore, MD, Williams & Wilkins, 1992, pp 79–113

Mattis S: Dementia Rating Scale. Odessa, FL, Psychological Assessment Resources, 1973

McKenna PJ, Tamlyn D, Lund CE, et al: Amnesic syndrome in schizophrenia. Psychol Med 20:967–972, 1990

Medalia A, Gold J, Merriam A: The effects of neuroleptics on neuropsychological tests results of schizophrenics. Archives of Clinical Neuropsychology 3:249–271, 1988

National Institute on Aging: Personnel for Health Needs of the Elderly Through Year 2020 (NIH Publ No 87-2950). Bethesda, MD, U.S. Department of Health and Human Services, 1987

Negrete JC, Knapp WP, Douglas DE, et al: Cannabis affects the severity of schizophrenic symptoms: results of a clinical survey. Psychol Med 16:515–520, 1986

Overall JE, Gorham DR: The Brief Psychiatric Rating Scale. Psychol Rep 10:799–812, 1962

Palmer BW, Heaton RK, Paulsen JP, et al: Schizophrenia patients with normal neurocognitive functioning: frequency and characteristics (abstract). Journal of the International Neuropsychology Society 2:55, 1996

Parsons OA, Butters N, Nathan PE: Neuropsychology of Alcoholism: Implications for Diagnosis and Treatment. New York, Guilford, 1987

Paulsen JS, Heaton RK, Sadek JR, et al: The nature of learning and memory impairments in schizophrenia. Journal of the International Neuropsychological Society 1:88–99, 1995

Perlick D, Mattis S, Stastny P, et al: Neuropsychological discriminators of long-term inpatient or outpatient status in chronic schizophrenia. J Neuropsychiatry Clin Neurosci 4:428–434, 1992

Physician's Desk Reference, 50th Edition. Montvale, NJ, Medical Economics Company, 1996

Powchik P, Davidson M, Nemeroff CB, et al: Alzheimer's-disease-related protein in geriatric schizophrenic patients with cognitive impairment. Am J Psychiatry 150:1726–1727, 1993

Prager S, Jeste DV: Sensory impairment in late-life schizophrenia. Schizophr Bull 19:755–772, 1993

Prohovnik I, Dwork AJ, Kaufman MA, et al: Alzheimer-type neuropathology in elderly schizophrenia patients. Schizophr Bull 19:805–816, 1993

Regier DA, Farmer ME, Rae DS, et al: Co-morbidity of mental disorders with alcohol and other drug abuse: results from the Epidemiologic Catchment Area (ECA) study. JAMA 264:2511–2518, 1990

Rice DP, Miller LS: The economic burden of schizophrenia: conceptual and methodological issues and cost estimates, in Handbook of Mental Health Economics and Health Policy, Vol 1: Schizophrenia. Edited by Moscarelli M, Rupp A. New York, Wiley, 1996, pp 321–334

Rovner BW, Steele CD, German P, et al: Psychiatric diagnosis and uncooperative behavior in nursing homes. J Geriatr Psychiatry Neurol 5:102–105, 1992

Royall DR, Mahurin RK, True JE, et al: Executive impairment among the functionally dependent: comparisons between schizophrenic and elderly subjects. Am J Psychiatry 150:1813–1819, 1993

Saykin AJ, Shtasel DL, Gur RE, et al: Neuropsychological deficits in neuroleptic naive patients with first-episode schizophrenia. Arch Gen Psychiatry 51:124–131, 1994

Schneider LS, Pollock VE, Lyness SA: A meta-analysis of controlled trials of neuroleptic treatment in dementia. J Am Geriatr Soc 38:553–563, 1990

Seltzer ML: The Michigan Alcohol Screening Test: the quest for a new diagnostic instrument. Am J Psychiatry 127:89–94, 1971

Silverstein ML, Zerwic MJ: Clinical psychopathologic symptoms in neuropsychologically impaired and intact schizophrenics. J Consult Clin Psychol 53:267–268, 1985

Skinner HA: The Drug Abuse Screening Test. Addict Behav 7:363–371, 1982

Soni SD, Mallik A: The elderly chronic schizophrenic inpatient: a study of psychiatric morbidity in 'elderly graduates.' Int J Geriatr Psychiatry 8:665–673, 1993

Spohn HE, Strauss ME: Relation of neuroleptic and anticholinergic medication to cognitive functions in schizophrenia. J Abnorm Psychol 98:367–380, 1989

Stephens JH, Ota KY, Carpenter WT, et al: Diagnostic criteria for schizophrenia, prognostic implications, and diagnostic overlap. Psychiatry Res 2:1–12, 1980

Stern Y, Sano M, Paulson J, et al: Modified Mini-Mental State Examination: validity and reliability. Neurology 37:179–186, 1987

Talbott JA, Linn L: Reactions of schizophrenics to life-threatening disease. Psychiatr Q 50:218–227, 1978

Thienhaus OJ, Allen A, Bennett JA, et al: Anticholinergic serum levels and cognitive performance. Eur Arch Psychiatry Clin Neurosci 240:28–33, 1990

Tollefson G, Montague-Clouse J, Lancaster SP: The relationship of serum anticholinergic activity to mental status performance in an elderly nursing home population. J Neuropsychiatry Clin Neurosci 3:314–319, 1991

Tune L, Coyle JT: Acute extrapyramidal side effects: serum levels of neuroleptics and anticholinergics. Psychopharmacology (Berl) 75:9–15, 1981

Tune L, Carr S, Hoag E, et al: Anticholinergic effects of drugs commonly prescribed for the elderly: potential means for assessing risk of delirium. Am J Psychiatry 149:1393–1394, 1992

Wisniewski HM, Constantinidis J, Wegiel J, et al: Neurofibrillary pathology in brains of elderly schizophrenics treated with neuroleptics. Alzheimer Dis Assoc Disord 8:211–227, 1994

Wyatt RJ, Henter I, Leary MC, et al: An economic evaluation of schizophrenia—1991. Soc Psychiatry Psychiatr Epidemiol 30:196–205, 1995

CHAPTER 8

Aggression and Violence in Patients With Schizophrenia

Leslie Citrome, M.D., M.P.H.
Jan Volavka, M.D., Ph.D.

Some patients diagnosed with schizophrenia are occasionally violent. This behavior endangers the safety of the patients themselves, their fellow patients, their families, and caregivers, mental health workers, and the general public.

Aggression may be defined as overt behavior involving intent to deliver noxious stimulation to another organism or to behave destructively toward inanimate objects. Humans evince three main subtypes of aggression: verbal aggression, physical aggression against other people, and physical aggression against objects. *Violence* usually denotes physical aggression against other people and thus can be seen as a subtype of aggression. *Crime* is an intentional violation of the criminal law committed without defense or excuse; the criminal intent cannot be formed without mental competence (hence the insanity defense). *Hostility* is a loosely defined term; in its various usages, it may include aggression, irritability, suspicion, uncooperativeness, and jealousy.

Portions of this chapter draw on Dr. Volavka's book *Neurobiology of Violence* (Washington, D.C., American Psychiatric Press, 1995).

We wish to acknowledge Menahem Krakowski, M.D., Ph.D., who contributed to the clinical vignettes.

Violent behavior in patients with schizophrenia can be categorized into violence in the community and violence in the hospital. In the community, patients with schizophrenia appear to be more likely to engage in violent behavior than persons without any diagnosed mental disorder, especially if they have a comorbid substance use disorder. Violent or threatening behavior is a frequent reason for admission to a psychiatric inpatient facility, and that behavior may continue after the admission.

Management of the violent patient diagnosed with schizophrenia begins with an assessment of the possible causes. The etiology of violent behavior in patients with schizophrenia is multifactorial:

1. Co-occurring substance abuse, dependence, and intoxication may facilitate violence (see Chapter 9, this volume).
2. The disease process itself may produce hallucinations and delusions that provoke violence.
3. Poor impulse control due to neuropsychiatric deficits may facilitate the discharge of aggressive tendencies.
4. Underlying character pathology may also influence the use of violent acts as a means to achieve certain goals.
5. The ward or other environment may be chaotic, further encouraging maladaptive behaviors.

The pattern of violent behavior may provide clues for management. The transiently violent and the persistently violent may differ in both the root cause for aggressivity and in the necessary ingredients for a successful treatment strategy.

Treatments include short-term sedation, mechanical restraints, preventive aggression devices, and placement in specialized and structured psychiatric intensive care units. Pharmacotherapy for the longer-term management of violent behavior is highly dependent on the individual patient's underlying clinical problem. Theoretical rationales for treatment strategies have included the serotonin hypothesis. The atypical antipsychotics (especially clozapine), beta-blockers, and mood stabilizers have been used with some success. Noncompliance with treatment can be an obstacle, especially in communities where outpatient commitment is not available.

Epidemiology of Violent Behavior in Patients With Schizophrenia

Behavior in the Community

Early prevalence estimates of violent behavior relied heavily on arrest records (Volavka 1995). If a suspect is apprehended, the police have considerable discretion in deciding whether to arrest and determining the charge. The discretionary power to adopt alternatives to arrest is typically exercised when suspects are juveniles or when they appear to be ill (in which case they may be taken to a hospital emergency room rather than to the police station). Even if an arrest is made, the charge may not fully reflect the severity of the criminal behavior. Arrest statistics thus underestimate the "true" crime rate and provide a biased description of offender characteristics as well as of the type of criminal behaviors actually occurring.

Data that are free from the biases of arrest statistics were obtained within the framework of the Epidemiologic Catchment Area (ECA) project. The primary purpose of the project was to estimate the prevalence of untreated psychiatric disorders in the population of the United States. To that end, structured diagnostic interviews were administered to more than 20,000 persons residing in five areas of the United States, either in the community or in institutions (Regier et al. 1990). In approximately 50% of this sample (i.e., approximately 10,000 persons), data on violence were fortuitously collected. The interviewers inquired about the following behaviors in the past year: use of a weapon in a fight, history of fighting, child beating, wife (or partner) beating, and physical fights while drinking. From this self-report, the subjects were dichotomously classified as either violent or nonviolent. A logistic regression model of predictors of violence was performed (Swanson 1994, p. 124). The predictors included gender, age, socioeconomic status, marital status, and psychiatric diagnosis. The effect of psychiatric diagnosis on the probability of being violent was computed after the effects of the other predictors were accounted for statistically (i.e., the other predictors were used as covariates). The resulting probability estimates for various diagnoses are displayed in Figure 8–1. As can be seen in the figure, the probabilities of violent behavior in male and female schizophrenia patients were, respectively, 5.3 times and 5.9 times higher than those in persons without any diagnosed mental disorder.

The results reported by Swanson were supported by a smaller epidemiological study that compared 385 psychiatric patients (current or former) living in a community with 365 residents of the same community

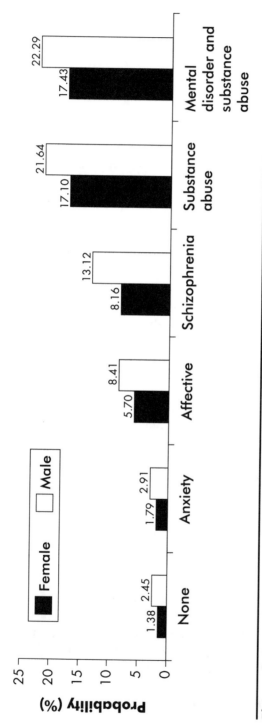

Figure 8–1. Predicted 1-year probability of violent behavior by sex and psychiatric diagnosis, as estimated by logistic regression.

Source. Reprinted with permission from Swanson JW: "Mental Disorder, Substance Abuse, and Community Violence: An Epidemiological Approach," in *Violence and Mental Disorder: Developments in Risk Assessment.* Edited by Monahan J, Steadman HJ. Chicago, IL, University of Chicago Press, 1994, pp. 101–136. Copyright 1994, University of Chicago Press.

who had never received psychiatric treatment (the number of subjects reported in this study varies slightly depending on the availability of data) (Link and Stueve 1994; Link et al. 1992). The self-reports of violent behaviors—hitting someone, fighting, and using a weapon—were, respectively, 2.4 times, 1.7 times, and 3.6 times more frequent in the patients than in the nonpatients (Link and Stueve 1994; see Table 2 of that publication). Interestingly, these violent behaviors were specifically related to three psychiatric symptoms: feeling of domination by external force, thought insertion, and feeling that people wished to harm the patient. The relevance of this study for schizophrenia is reduced by the fact that only 19.4% of the patients had this diagnosis.

A study of an unselected Swedish birth cohort ($N = 15,117$) (Hodgins 1992) supported and expanded the relationships reported above. Men with major mental disorders were approximately four times more likely to have been convicted of a violent offense than men without any mental disorder, and women were approximately 27 times more likely to be convicted than women without any mental disorder. A larger unselected cohort comprising 324,401 Danes (Hodgins et al. 1996) revealed that both men and women hospitalized at least once with mental disorders were more likely to have registered for at least one violent crime than persons with no history of psychiatric admissions.

Some of the violent behavior occurring among schizophrenic patients is attributable to comorbidity with substance abuse (Lindqvist and Allebeck 1990; Swanson 1994). The relationship is illustrated in Figure 8–1, which shows that substance abuse increases the probability of violent behavior substantially more than schizophrenia alone, and is supported by a number of epidemiological studies. An Australian case linkage study (Wallace et al. 1998) found 70 patients with schizophrenia who had been convicted of a serious crime out of a cohort of 4,156 persons. There was a strong interaction between mental disorder and substance abuse. For men, the odds ratio for violent offenses jumped from 2.4 ($P < 0.001$) for individuals with schizophrenia without substance abuse to 18.8 ($P < 0.001$) for individuals with schizophrenia complicated by substance abuse. A report from Finland revealed that although the risk of committing a homicide was about 10 times greater for schizophrenia patients than it was in the general population, the risk increased to greater than 17 times for male patients with schizophrenia and coexisting alcoholism and more than 80 times for female patients with schizophrenia and coexisting alcoholism (Eronen et al. 1996). These findings are consistent with those from another Finnish study of an unselected birth cohort ($N = 11,017$) (Rasanen et al. 1998), in which men who abused alcohol and were diagnosed with schizophrenia were found to be 25.2 (95% confidence interval [CI] = 6.1, 97.5) times more likely to commit violent crimes than mentally healthy men. However, the risk for nonalcoholic patients with schizophrenia was 3.6 (95% CI = 0.9, 12.3), indicating that statistical significance was not reached for this group ($P = 0.06$). It should be noted that these estimates were based on small numbers of subjects: there were 11 patients with schizophrenia and comorbid alcoholism, 4 of whom were violent offenders, and 40 patients with schizophrenia but no alcoholism, 3 of whom were violent offenders (Rasanen et al. 1998; see Table 1 of that publication).

Similar results regarding the influence of substance abuse were found in a recent prospective study of 1,136 psychiatric patients in the United States (Steadman et al. 1998). No significant difference was found between the 1-year prevalence of violence by patients without symptoms of substance abuse (4.3%) and by community control subjects (3.3%), who also were free of symptoms of substance abuse. Substance abuse symptoms significantly increased the rate of violence to 14.1% of the patient sample and to 11.1% of the control group. However, questions remain regarding the methodology of the study (see Czobor and Volavka 1999), including the possibility that the study did not account for patients who may be repeatedly assaultive and whose condition is treatment resistant and who are lost to follow-up.

History of violent behavior and schizophrenia in different cultures was the focus of a World Health Organization (WHO) study (Volavka et al. 1997). The occurrence rate of assault in the cohort of 1,017 patients with schizophrenia was 20.6%, with the rate three times higher in developing countries (Colombia, India, Nigeria) (31.5%) compared with developed countries (Denmark, Ireland, Japan, United Kingdom, United States, and the former countries of Czechoslovakia and the U.S.S.R.) (10.5%). The difference between the developing and the developed countries in the rate of history of assault remained significant even when demographic, alcohol/drug use, and base crime rate variables were considered.

Thus, these epidemiological studies demonstrate an elevated probability of violent behavior among psychiatric patients, especially when a comorbid substance use disorder is present. However, a causal relationship between violence and psychosis has not been established by these studies. Support for a hypothesis stating that psychosis causes violence would require a finding of a clear temporal linkage between them; one would also need to test whether the patients are more violent when they are more psychotic.

That linkage was studied by interviewing 121 incarcerated psychotic forensic patients about the motives for the offenses committed while they were living in the community (Taylor 1985). Most of these patients were diagnosed with schizophrenia. The author estimated that 82% of their offenses (violent and nonviolent offenses combined) were attributable to their illness. Delusions were the driving force for violent offending among these patients. Thus, this study established the time linkage between delusions and the offense that was lacking in the studies discussed earlier in this section (Link and Stueve 1994; Link et al. 1992; Swanson 1994): the patients were delusional at the time they committed their offenses.

Data from the ECA project and other more recent studies discussed above represent a major advance in the epidemiology of violent behavior in individuals with schizophrenia. However, they have certain weaknesses. One of these weaknesses is that violent behaviors (e.g., fighting) are presented as categorical variables (present or absent). Thus, recidivistically violent patients are lumped together with those who are violent just once. Frequency of violent behavior is an important variable. Persistent (recidivistic) and transient violence may differ in their neurobiological underpinning, management, and social consequences.

Behavior in the Hospital

Short-Term Hospitalization

Violent or threatening behavior is a frequent reason for admission to a psychiatric inpatient facility, and that behavior may continue after the admission. The association between preadmission threats and postadmission violence is particularly strong among schizophrenia patients (McNiel and Binder 1989). During the first 24 hours after the admission to a psychiatric inpatient unit, 33 of 253 patients (13.0%) physically attacked another person (Binder and McNiel 1988). A subset of this sample consisted of patients diagnosed with schizophrenia (N = 87); 9 of these patients (10.3%) attacked another person during the same period. Another group reported that in the first 8 days after hospitalization, 25 of 289 patients with schizophrenia or schizoaffective disorder (8.7%) assaulted someone at least once (Tanke and Yesavage 1985).

Long-Term Hospitalization

A study of 5,164 long-term patients indicated that 7% of these patients physically attacked another person at least once during a 3-month period (Tardiff and Sweillam 1982). A subset of this sample consisted of patients diagnosed with schizophrenia (N = 3,294); 232 of these patients (7%) attacked another person during the same period (Tardiff and Sweillam 1982; see Table 1 of that publication).

This and similar studies do not distinguish between recidivistic and transient assaultiveness. But, as noted earlier, such a distinction is important. A 6-month study of 1,552 inpatients with various diagnoses detected 576 violent incidents; a small group of recidivistic patients (5%) caused 53% of the incidents (Convit et al. 1990). The diagnosis of schizophrenia was slightly overrepresented among the male recidivists; personality and impulse disorder diagnoses were frequent among both the male and female recidivists. A 7-month study of 174 inpatients in Australia provided similar information (Owen et al. 1998a). The recidivistic patients (12%) accounted for 69% of the 752 violent incidents identified. The male recidivists were more likely to have an organic brain syndrome, and the women recidivists were more likely to have a personality disorder.

Patient Assessment and Differential Diagnosis

Acute Episode Versus Chronic Pattern of Aggressive Behavior

Patient assessment involves gathering information about past and current behavior from the patient, providers of health care, family and friends, a review of past treatment (both successful and unsuccessful), and a clinical examination of the patient over time. Laboratory and neuropsychiatric testing, as well as neuroimaging, would help round out the assessment. A differential diagnosis could then be formulated and a treatment strategy could be crafted.

In the assessment of the acutely agitated patient whose history is unknown, attempts are made to rule out somatic conditions that require emergency treatment. Delirium is a medical emergency. Once the patient is under behavioral control, further medical and psychiatric workups can be done. Mechanical restraints may be necessary to prevent the agitated patient from injuring himself or herself or others while the medical workup is being conducted.

For the acutely agitated patient in whom the episode is one of many, the acute episode is managed and then strategies are designed to reduce their intensity and frequency. Later in this chapter we discuss in detail treatment approaches and options for acute agitation and chronic aggressivity.

For the patient diagnosed with schizophrenia, care must be taken not to miss comorbid conditions such as alcohol or sedative abuse or dependence that may be accompanied by acute intoxication or withdrawal. Concomitant seizure disorder may further complicate the clinical picture, in particular if neuroleptic therapy appears to worsen the condition. Adverse drug effects such as akathisia may serve as a stimulus for striking out (Keckich 1978; Siris 1985). Antisocial personality traits may be the most important factor in some instances of patient violence in which goal-directed behavior such as extortion of money or cigarettes is present.

Assessment Instruments

Aggressivity and hostility can be assessed with general scales such as the Minnesota Multiphasic Personality Inventory (MMPI), which has been used in studies of violent behavior (Lothstein and Jones 1978; Rogers and Seman 1983). The MMPI has been combined with neuropsychological testing to successfully discriminate between violent and nonviolent male inmates (Spellacy 1978). Researchers have used scales such as the Buss-Durkee Hostility Inventory (Buss and Durkee 1957), the Brown-Goodwin Inventory (Brown et al. 1979), the Albert Einstein College of Medicine Past Feelings and Acts of Violence Scale (Plutchik and Van Praag 1990; Plutchik et al. 1989), and the Overt Aggression Scale (Silver and Yudofsky 1991; Yudofsky et al. 1986).

Standard official documentation of aggressive incidents varies from facility to facility but can serve as a valuable source of information in assessing a patient's clinical status. Official documents may underreport incidents (Convit et al. 1988; Lion et al. 1981). Review of prescribed "as needed" (prn) medication use may provide clues about the degree of agitation experienced by the patient and observed by the staff.

Risk Assessment

Basics in risk assessment include determining past history of violence, evaluating current access to weapons, and asking about violent ideation. Criminal justice records are another means of assessing past history and recently have been made available to the providers of care in New York State psychiatric hospitals. Protecting the therapist from breaching the duty to protect (the so-called Tarasoff liability) has been one focus of risk assessment (Monahan 1993).

The prediction of violence has been a particularly nettlesome problem in forensic psychiatry. A study of correlates of accuracy in the assessment of psychiatric inpatients' risk of violence examined diagnosis, mental status, history of violence, and demographic variables (McNiel and Binder 1995). The accuracy of the prediction of high risk for violence was enhanced when the diagnosis was schizophrenia. Past history of violence is probably the best single predictor of violence (Blomhoff et al. 1990; Convit et al. 1988; Karson and Bigelow 1987). Wartime combat experience in patients with schizophrenia can also serve as a predictor for dangerous behavior, more so than premorbid criminal behavior (Yesavage 1983a, 1983b). In one study, it was demonstrated that gender is not a strong predictor of involvement in violence by psychiatric patients (Newhill et al. 1995). However, this study included all patients seen in a psychiatric emergency service where only 7% of females and 9% of males were categorized as having schizophrenia or schizoaffective disorder.

A paranoid schizophrenia patient with a delusional focus on interpersonal relationships may be sufficiently intact to actually plan and execute violent acts (Krakowski et al. 1986), but the presence of paranoid delusions in itself may not predict violence (Calcedo-Barba and Calcedo-Ordonez 1994). The role of paranoid delusions in predicting violence has been a focus in the prevention of violence in the workplace (Boxer 1993), in which paranoid schizophrenia, delusional disorder, and paranoid personality disorder are considered. Those who make threats toward the president of the United States or other prominent American political figures are typically described as having chronic paranoid schizophrenia (Shore et al. 1988). A recent report on delusions and symptom-consistent violence among 54 hospitalized patients (of which 28 were diagnosed with schizophrenia) in Louisiana (Junginger et al. 1998) concluded that most violent incidents are not motivated by concurrent delusions but that some may be: a small subgroup of violent subjects (17.5%) reported at least one incident that was judged to be both extremely violent and definitely motivated by a concurrent delusion. This is consistent with the finding of an association between increased risk for violence and persecutory delusions (Cheung et al. 1997). Examining the phenomenology of delusions in more detail may assist in risk assessment (Buchanan 1997).

Differentiating Patterns of Violence

Central to the development of a differential diagnosis is the analysis of the pattern of violence. The nature of the aggressive episodes—whether they are singular or repetitive, regular or sporadic, or with low or high potential of actual injury—will guide the clinician in formulating immediate management plans, provisional diagnosis, and long-term strategy.

Some patients are transiently violent when in a chaotic environment, whereas others are persistently violent no matter how stable the environment is (Krakowski and Czobor 1997). Persistently violent patients were found to be more likely to have neurological impairments, as evidenced by impairments in stereognosis, graphesthesia, tandem walk, and walking-associated movements, and selective impairment in visual-spatial functioning on neuropsychological testing (Krakowski et al. 1989a, 1989b). In another study, lateralized abnormalities on electroencephalograms (EEGs) were found in a group of persistently violent psychiatric inpatients, most of whom had schizophrenia (Convit et al. 1991). Organic brain dysfunction has been found in maximum-security forensic psychiatric patients (Martell 1992). A quantified neurological examination has been developed to assess subtle neurological dysfunction and was found to differentiate violent from matched nonviolent psychiatric inpatients (Convit et al. 1988). This exam has also been related to the degree of violence and to treatment response (Krakowski et al. 1989b). In one study, brain computed tomography was used to compare violent and nonviolent schizophrenia inpatients (Convit et al. 1996), but the results of this pilot study did not demonstrate any significant differences other than a possibly larger Sylvian fissure for the violent group. A more detailed discussion of the neurology of aggression in general can be found elsewhere (Hamstra 1986; Weiger and Bear 1988), as can reviews of the psychobiology of the violent offender (Volavka et al. 1992) and the neurobiology of violence (Volavka 1995).

In contrast to persistently violent patients, patients who were transiently violent were more likely to respond to a new structured environment (Krakowski et al. 1988). Environmental factors that lead to increased aggressive behavior on a psychiatric ward include crowding (Palmstierna et al. 1991) and possibly an overly authoritative attitude by nursing staff and underinvolvement of medical staff with ward activities (Brailsford and Stevenson 1973). Time of day may be a factor, with a peak problem period of 7:00 A.M. to 9:00 A.M. reported in one facility (Fottrell 1980). Other environmental factors found to increase the risk of violent incidents include more staff without psychiatric training or aggression training, more nonnursing staff on planned leave, more students on the ward, and, paradoxically, more nursing staff on duty (either men or women), including more senior nurses on duty (Owen et al. 1998b). Possible explanations for the last mentioned include increased stimulation and limit setting and more staff to notice and record more violent incidents. It appears that transiently violent patients are more responsive to typical neuroleptic medication and have less neurological impairment than persistently violent patients (Volavka and Krakowski 1989).

Differential Diagnosis

Patients with schizophrenia living in the community are not usually persistently violent, but they may present acutely with aggressive and violent behavior. Their behavior may be due to acute decompensation secondary to covert or overt noncompliance with psychotropic medication. Decompensation may also be due to a failure of the current medication regimen. Blood levels of neuroleptics were found to be inversely correlated with danger-related events in a group of recently hospitalized male schizophrenic patients (Yesavage 1982). Studies report that from 24% to 44% of aggressive incidents committed by individuals with schizophrenia occur during an acute phase of the illness (Beaudoin et al. 1993; Humphreys et al. 1992; Virkkunen 1974). The clinical features expected would be a worsening of psychotic symptoms and possibly command hallucinations. Patients with schizophrenia and violent behavior, compared with patients with schizophrenia without violent behavior, were reported to be more likely to experience persecutory delusions and auditory hallucinations that make them feel sad, angry, anxious, and intruded upon (Cheung et al. 1997). No associations were found between violent behavior and command hallucinations, although the importance of this in violent behavior is in dispute (Humphreys et al. 1992; Junginger 1995; McNiel 1994; Rogers et al. 1988).

Substance Abuse

The epidemiological studies described earlier demonstrate that patients with both schizophrenia and a substance use disorder are at much higher risk of violent behavior than patients with schizophrenia alone. The combination of substance abuse and nonadherence to a medication regimen is of particular concern (Swartz et al. 1998). Schizophrenia and substance use disorders co-occur more frequently than would be expected by chance. Data from the ECA project discussed earlier indicate that 47% of all individuals with a lifetime diagnosis of schizophrenia have also met the criteria for substance abuse or dependence (Regier et al. 1990). Schizophrenia was found to elevate very significantly the risks for alcohol dependence and drug dependence. Conversely, substance use disorders elevated the risk for schizophrenia. Aggressive and violent behavior in patients with schizophrenia can be precipitated by alcohol, cocaine, phencyclidine (PCP), or amphetamine intoxication (Smith and Hucker 1994). The importance of these findings is underscored by the reported increase in the prevalence estimates of comorbid substance abuse with schizophrenia over several decades (Cuffel 1992).

Substance abuse among those arrested is common: cocaine has been detected in the urine of male arrestees at rates ranging from 16% in San Jose, California, to 59% in Atlanta, Georgia (Maguire and Pastore 1997; see Table 4.31 of that publication). Odds of violence are particularly elevated among patients with schizophrenia or schizoaffective disorder who also exhibit a pattern of polysubstance abuse (Cuffel et al. 1994). Inpatients can also be abusing illicit substances because access to drugs and alcohol, although difficult, is not impossible. Caffeine intoxication, water intoxication, antihistamine intoxication, as well as the ingestion of deodorants and aerosols, have also been described among inpatients (Koczapski et al. 1990).

Medical Conditions

Medical conditions such as newly developed brain tumors or metabolic disturbances may precipitate aggressive behavior in a patient not normally known to be violent. For patients already in the hospital, regular and routine physical assessments that include laboratory tests can be expected to screen out most problems.

For patients with a history of seizure disorder, evidence suggests that interictal violence is associated more with psychopathology and mental retardation than with epileptiform activity or other seizure variables (Mendez et al. 1993).

Antisocial Personality Disorder

Antisocial personality disorders may coexist with schizophrenia, and antisocial personality traits may be present even if the full disorder cannot be diagnosed. Data from the ECA project indicate that in males diagnosed with antisocial personality disorder, schizophrenia occurs at a rate 7 times higher (and in females, 12 times higher) than the expected rate (Robins et al. 1991, pp. 288–289). These strong cross-sectional associations between schizophrenia and antisocial personality disorder are consistent with the observation of frequent conduct problems in the premorbid history of schizophrenic patients (Robins 1966, p. 240). A co-occurring antisocial personality disorder in a patient with schizophrenia increases the risk of severe substance abuse, psychiatric impairment, aggression, and legal problems (Mueser et al. 1997).

Violence occurring in patients with schizophrenia and antisocial personality disorder or traits may be evaluated by examining the context of the aggressive incident. Intimidation of patients and staff or material gain may be factors. For example, there may be fighting over money, cigarettes, or access to sexual partners, and attacks on caregivers who deny a patient's request or try to set limits to patients' behavior (e.g., enforcing a smoking ban). Engagement in illegal activities, rule breaking, lying, and a lack of remorse are only a few of the criteria in the diagnosis of antisocial personality disorder in DSM-IV (American Psychiatric Association 2000).

These characteristics may be found in both inpatient and outpatient populations. Misdiagnosis of schizophrenia as antisocial personality disorder can occur, possibly leading to a missed opportunity for treatment (Travin and Protter 1982). Chronically psychotic patients can also make sociopathic adaptations to the environments imposed on them as a result of their illnesses, and this can distort the clinical picture; an example is when an individual's psychotic symptoms diminish when his welfare check is due to arrive (Geller 1980).

Diagnostic Procedures

No laboratory diagnostic procedures for schizophrenia are available, but research demonstrates interesting findings in this regard. Neurochemical, neurological, neuropsychological, and electrophysiological correlates of violent behavior are being actively investigated (Volavka 1995). At present it may be helpful for the purposes of prognostication and long-term treatment planning to tease apart the persistently violent from the transiently violent. An assessment of neurological functioning like that described earlier, including neuropsychological testing, may be useful.

> David is a 33-year-old man who was diagnosed as having schizophrenia when he was first hospitalized at age 21. He presented this time to the emergency room with auditory hallucinations of a male voice's commenting on his actions, and the delusion that the FBI had been keeping him under surveillance. His compliance with his prescribed regimen of haloperidol was considered very doubtful. While waiting to be admitted to the psychiatric inpatient unit, he became increasingly agitated, stating he was being harassed by the FBI. He was administered lorazepam 2 mg orally, in addition to being restarted on his regular regimen of haloperidol 10 mg twice daily. Once on the ward he continued to be agitated and subsequently hit a fellow patient in the face, stating afterward that he believed the victim was a federal agent assigned to destroy him. David was transferred to the psychiatric intensive care unit (PICU), where he was convinced that he would be safe from harm. After 8 days of steady improvement, he appeared to be in good behavioral control and was returned to the regular ward, where the environment was more chaotic, with several more patients in a small geographic space and fewer staff than on the PICU. Almost immediately, David struck another patient and was returned to intensive care. David remained on the PICU for another 3 weeks before being discharged back to his family.

The scenario above illustrates several points: First, David was initially acutely psychotic with prominent paranoid delusions. He struck a patient while under the influence of these delusions. He was able to regain behavioral control after several days of resuming his antipsychotic medication.

Second, When David was returned to the regular unit, the environment was more chaotic and he struck another patient. This time the actual motive was unclear, because the intensity of his paranoid delusions was significantly less than on admission to the hospital. Thus, we have an example of a transiently violent patient whose initial aggression was determined by his psychotic symptoms but who became violent again when exposed to the environmental stressor of a less structured treatment setting.

John is a 55-year-old man receiving care on a long-term care unit of a state hospital whose condition meets the DSM-IV criteria for chronic schizophrenia, undifferentiated type. John has been intermittently agitated, striking other patients with his closed fist. He has been unable to provide any reason for his behavior. Attempts to decrease the frequency of his outbursts by increasing his dose of antipsychotic medication (chlorpromazine) have failed. Even upon his many transfers to the secure care unit, he continued to be unpredictably assaultive and frequently required the application of mechanical restraints. A visiting neuropsychologist suggested a specialized workup at the affiliated university hospital. Although John did not show any physical signs of coarse brain disease, subtle neuropsychological deficits were suspected. John was administered the Wisconsin Card Sorting Test, and he demonstrated perseveration in classifying items: he was not able to modify his pattern of classification when provided with new information. [This test is related to dorsolateral prefrontal cerebral cortex function, and neuropsychological abnormalities in this area can be seen in many patients with schizophrenia (Weinberger et al. 1986).] John was also evaluated on the Quantified Neurological Scale (Convit et al. 1994), which revealed impairment on frontal motor tasks.

The vignette above demonstrates a patient who is persistently violent and has subtle neurological deficits. This conclusion led to the consideration of more novel pharmacological approaches, including the use of both valproic acid and carbamazepine, which decreased the number of violent incidents over time but unfortunately did not eliminate them entirely. The patient is currently undergoing a trial of clozapine.

Henry is a 30-year-old man who has spent most of the past 12 years in psychiatric hospitals or halfway houses. He has also spent some time in local jails and in the forensic psychiatric hospital after committing various minor crimes. Henry has been diagnosed with paranoid schizophrenia, antisocial personality traits, and intermittent alcohol abuse. His most recent stay in the halfway house was for the most part uneventful. Henry took his antipsychotic medication, attended the group meetings, and appeared to be doing satisfactorily. One evening he went to the local tavern and consumed enough alcohol to appear visibly inebriated and was asked to leave after getting into a loud argument with the bartender. Upon his return to the halfway house, he proceeded to beat his roommate, accusing him of controlling his thoughts. He was subsequently readmitted to the local community hospital where the emergency room staff appeared to be most familiar with him, telling the on-call psychiatrist that Henry had been admitted many times under similar circumstances.

The case example above illustrates the interplay among schizophrenia, alcohol abuse, and antisocial personality traits. Henry was disinhibited because of the influence of alcohol intoxication. This led to his acting out on his chronic paranoid delusions. It is noted that in the past he had frequently resorted to fighting and that he did not follow rules well. In general, alcohol or substance abuse may be the trigger for violent decompensation. As shown in Figure 8–1, the probability of violent behavior is higher for persons with both a mental disorder and substance abuse. Efforts to reduce and eliminate the comorbid abuse disorder are critical in reducing aggressive behavior and violence in this population.

Treatment

General Behavioral Management of Acute Aggression

A number of books and articles offer good practical advice on handling agitated patients and training issues (Citrome and Green 1990; Eichelman and Hartwig 1995; Gertz 1980; Lehmann et al. 1983; Tardiff 1992; Thackrey 1987; Tupin 1983). Others focus on restraint and seclusion (Fisher 1994) and psychodynamic strategies (Gibson 1967). A comprehensive biopsychosocial approach, involving the multidisciplinary team, is key in optimally managing crisis situations. Organizations such as NAPPI (Non-Abusive Psychological and Physical Intervention, Inc.) are available to train hospital and clinic staff in methods of assessing, preventing, and physically managing dangerous behavior (Lalemand 1998). Typically, the staff is trained as a team and includes physicians, nurses, therapy aides, social workers, psychologists, security personnel, and any other people who might have patient contact.

Clinicians are urged to survey the environment for potential weapons, not to turn their back on the patient, and to have other staff available. Taking verbal threats seriously and being aware of physical premonitory signs such as a clenched fist and pacing are important. Training staff in crisis management is a priority in many facilities as a means to reduce staff and patient injury.

In any emergency, treatment options are limited to those that are immediately effective and that interfere the least with the patient's physical and mental well-being. Initially, an aggressive patient should be isolated from other patients and from distractions, because extraneous stimulation can intensify psychosis in a patient who may be hallucinating, paranoid, and agitated. Moreover, other patients may intentionally or inadvertently interfere with treatment. Generally, it is easier to clear the area of many calm patients than to move one dangerous individual. Verbal interventions designed to calm patients include demonstrating empathy (Lane 1986) and providing a relaxed and confident demeanor from which the patient can model, all in the presence of many staff who stand by. Restraint or seclusion may be necessary, and it is during this process that the risk for injury for both staff and patients is highest. The technique of the calming blanket, a soft comforter with canvas reinforcements, may be helpful in subduing the patient who is punching, scratching, or kicking.

There is no specific pharmacological treatment for violent or aggressive behavior; however, nonspecific sedation is often used in the management of an acutely agitated patient. In general, intramuscular injection of a sedative has a faster onset of action than oral administration, but it has been observed that a patient may calm down readily after an oral dose, knowing that action has been taken and help is being provided. Sublingual administration may have a faster onset of action than oral ingestion and has the added advantage of distracting the agitated patient while the pill is dissolving.

Lorazepam appears to be a sound and rational choice when treating a patient experiencing an acute episode of agitation (Salzman 1988), especially when the etiology of the agitation is not clear. Lorazepam is a nonspecific sedating agent of the benzodiazepine class. Of all the benzodiazepines available, lorazepam is the only one reliably absorbed when administered intramuscularly (Greenblatt et al. 1979, 1982). Its half-life is relatively short (10–20 hours), and its route of elimination produces no active metabolites. The usual dosage of 0.5–2.0 mg every 1–6 hours may be administered orally, sublingually, intramuscularly, or intravenously. Caution is required when respiratory depression is a possibility, but this is less of a problem than with sodium Amytal (Tupin 1983), a sedating agent that was frequently used for this indication before the advent of lorazepam. There have been reports of an interaction between benzodiazepines and clozapine, producing (sometimes fatal) respiratory depression (Friedman et al. 1991; Klimke and Klieser 1994) and marked sedation, excessive sialorrhea, and ataxia (Cobb et al. 1991), but this combination has been used successfully by a number of practitioners (Kanofsky and Lindenmayer 1993).

Lorazepam is not recommended for long-term daily use because of the problems associated with tolerance, dependence, and withdrawal. Paradoxical reactions to benzodiazepines, as exhibited by hostility or violence, have been an area of concern (Bond and Lader 1979), but the evidence is not convincing. In any event, disinhibition with benzodiazepines is uncommon (Dietch and Jennings 1988) and is even more unlikely to occur when given within the context of single or limited doses in a crisis situation (Volavka 1995).

The possibility of alcohol or sedative withdrawal as a cause of agitation is another point in favor of using lorazepam. The use of a neuroleptic in this instance is suboptimal and may lower the seizure threshold. If delirium tremens is present, full supportive medical care must be available; when medical complications arise, the mortality rate may be as high as 20% (Victor 1966).

Neuroleptics universally cause sedation, given a high enough dose. Haloperidol, a butyrophenone, has been frequently used as an intramuscular prn medication for agitation and aggressive behavior (Clinton et al. 1987). It has been used in an emergency department setting for a wide variety of patients (Clinton et al. 1987). The advantages of haloperidol over the low-potency neuroleptics (e.g., chlorpromazine) are that it causes less hypotension, fewer anticholinergic side effects, and less of a decrease in the seizure threshold. Despite these advantages of haloperidol over chlorpromazine, clinicians may desire a more sedating agent, and so the low-potency neuroleptics continue to be used. In addition to this nonspecific sedation, a benefit of a neuroleptic would be its antipsychotic effect, but this would be evident only after the acute episode of agitation has subsided. Although once popular, rapid tranquilization with injectable haloperidol (Donlon et al. 1979) does not lead to a more extensive or rapid alleviation of psychotic symptoms (Neborsky et al. 1981), as observed in a group of mainly schizophrenia patients. Neuroleptics may have a longer-lasting effect on the reduction of agitation by treating the underlying psychosis. On the other hand, high doses of neuroleptics may lead to more adverse effects, including akathisia, and, as noted earlier, akathisia itself may provoke violent behavior (Keckich 1978; Siris 1985). For patients with conditions that are treatment resistant to typical neuroleptics, there are no benefits beyond the acute sedative effect.

Droperidol, another neuroleptic in the butyrophenone class, is used most often for induction of anesthesia. The medication is not approved by the Food and Drug Administration (FDA) for psychiatric conditions, but it has been used for sedating agitated patients in an emergency room setting (Thomas et al. 1992). A case report of coma following intravenous droperidol given for post-ECT delirium is cautionary (Koo and Chien 1986), and adequate medical backup and the availability of intubation and oxygen are urged (Schatzberg and Cole 1991). Thus, droperidol should not be used in psychiatric hospitals where such backup is not immediately available.

The new atypical antipsychotics may emerge as important options in the management of acute agitation in psychosis. Although sedation remains the primary mode of action when the atypical antipsychotics are used emergently for the acutely agitated patient, these agents have several advantages over typical antipsychotics (Citrome 1997). The advantages include a lower propensity for extrapyramidal side effects, including akathisia; a lower propensity for inducing tardive dyskinesia; and perhaps a specific antiaggressive effect over time, as will be described later. A current limitation is the lack of FDA-approved intramuscular preparations of atypical antipsychotics. This may change upon the possible approval of ziprasidone. Intramuscular ziprasidone has been studied in acutely agitated patients in Phase III clinical trials with some success in reducing the symptoms of agitation, with no or little resultant dystonia or akathisia (Reeves et al. 1998a, 1998b; Swift et al. 1998). Whether ziprasidone has specific antiaggressive properties in the same manner as clozapine (described below) remains unknown.

Longer-Term Management

Once the acute agitation is managed, longer-term strategies are required. As useful as lorazepam is as an acute intervention, it is not recommended as a long-term solution. Specialized units such as secure or psychiatric intensive care units (Citrome et al. 1995; Goldney et al. 1985; Musisi et al. 1989; Warneke 1986) provide a structured environment that optimizes staff and patient safety. In general, these specialized units are staffed with persons trained in interacting with volatile and difficult-to-manage patients (Maier et al. 1987).

Preventive aggression devices (referred to as PADS) are a form of ambulatory restraints that can be used as an alternative to seclusion (Van Rybroek et al. 1987). The technique was first developed for a specialized inpatient unit with repetitively aggressive patients. Patients in these wrist-to-belt and/or ankle-ankle restraints can remain with their peers on the ward, eat their meals, and interact, yet are prevented from striking out and injuring others. In combination with a comprehensive behavior modification program, these patients can be weaned off the use of the ambulatory restraints.

Pharmacotherapy for the Prevention of Aggressive Behavior in Patients With Schizophrenia

Treatment of the underlying disorder is key. Unfortunately, perhaps one-third of patients with schizophrenia either do not respond to antipsychotic treatment or respond only partially (Volavka 1995). Chronically violent patients with schizophrenia may receive higher doses of neuroleptics without clear evidence that such a regimen reduces the incidence of violent behavior (Krakowski et al. 1993).

The serotonergic system is involved in the modulation of aggressive behavior in many species, and a disturbance of this system has been implicated in impulsive violence in humans. Impulsive violent behavior may be directed against others or against self (Apter et al. 1990; Roy and Linnoila 1988). These issues have been extensively reviewed elsewhere (Virkkunen et al. 1995; Volavka 1995). In humans, disturbance of the serotonergic system has been inferred from low levels of 5-hydroxyindoleacetic acid (5-HIAA) in the cerebrospinal fluid (CSF) (Linnoila et al. 1983; Virkkunen and Linnoila 1990; Virkkunen et al. 1989, 1995) or from a blunted response to neuroendocrine challenges (Coccaro et al. 1989). This work was done largely with aggressive patients not with schizophrenia, but with personality disorders and substance use disorders.

Atypical Antipsychotics

The role of the serotonergic system in the pathogenesis of schizophrenia recently has received increased research attention. The interest in this topic has been stimulated by the success of atypical antipsychotics that have serotonergic effects (clozapine and risperidone). A large body of research is focusing on interactions between the serotonergic and the dopaminergic systems in schizophrenia (Kapur and Remington 1996). Nevertheless, little information on the serotonergic system and its functioning in aggressive patients with schizophrenia is available. The currently used probes of the serotonergic function in humans, such as CSF 5-HIAA assays and neuroendocrine challenges, yield results that can be distorted by concomitant medication, including antipsychotics. Medications usually can be safely discontinued for weeks or months in patients who are not currently very aggressive and psychotic; such patients (e.g., those with personality disorders) served as subjects in most studies linking the serotonergic system and aggression. However, discontinuation of antipsychotics may be seen as risky in violent schizophrenia patients. This problem has probably contributed to the lack of data on serotonin and aggression in schizophrenia. The CSF levels of 5-HIAA in a small sample of aggressive schizophrenia patients ($N = 10$) were not different from those obtained in a group of matched control subjects (Kunz et al. 1995). In this study, the authors were unable to discontinue antipsychotic treatment of the subjects for an adequate period of time; this problem may have contributed to the negative result. However, in spite of the lack of specific information on the role of serotonin in aggression among individuals with schizophrenia, the serotonin hypothesis has been a theoretical mainstay of the treatment of aggression in patients with this disorder.

Clozapine. The atypical antipsychotic clozapine, in addition to being an effective treatment in patients with conditions refractory to typical neuroleptics, may have specific antiaggressive effects. These effects may be due to its effects on the serotonergic system as well as its selective affinity for the limbic system (Volavka 1995). One retrospective study in a state hospital found that the number of violent episodes among schizophrenia inpatients decreased after they began clozapine treatment (Wilson and Claussen 1995). Similar results were found among five schizophrenia patients on a specialized unit for the severely aggressive (Ratey et al. 1993).

In a program spanning 21 state hospitals in New York State, 223 patients with schizophrenia who were receiving clozapine were assessed with the Brief Psychiatric Rating Scale (BPRS) at baseline, 6 weeks, 12 weeks, and at the end point. A selective effect of clozapine on hostility was found (Volavka et al. 1993). Another study reported a reduction in the use of seclusion and restraint in a group of patients with schizophrenia or schizoaffective disorder who were receiving clozapine in a state hospital (Chiles et al. 1994). This reduction in the use of restraints and seclusion was also observed among 107 "chronic" patients in state hospitals in Missouri after they began receiving clozapine (Mallya et al. 1992).

Buckley et al. (1995), in their report of 11 patients with schizophrenia who were treated with clozapine, suggested that because the magnitude of the reduction in aggression (again measured by the use of restraints and seclusion) was greater than the modest improvement noted in BPRS scores, clozapine had a selective antiaggressive effect. Other studies have demonstrated similar effects (Spivak et al. 1997), which have allowed patients to be transferred to less secure units and/or to achieve higher levels of patient privileges (Ebrahim et al. 1994; Maier 1992). Although no controlled studies of the antiaggressive effects of clozapine are yet available, the preponderance of evidence indicates that this drug reduces aggressive behavior in patients with schizophrenia and schizoaffective disorder (Glazer and Dickson 1998; Volavka and Citrome 1999). These effects cannot be fully explained by sedation or by general antipsychotic effects.

Risperidone. The atypical neuroleptic risperidone also has effects on the serotonergic system and was demonstrated to have a selective effect on hostility as well (Czobor et al. 1995). The authors had access to the database generated by the 9-week multicenter double-blind, placebo-controlled parallel group clinical trial of risperidone versus haloperidol (Marder and Meibach 1994). Hostility was measured by the Positive and Negative Syndrome Scale. Of the total sample, 139 patients had a baseline hostility score of at least mild, and all these patients carried the diagnosis of schizophrenia. Risperidone was found to have a greater selective effect on hostility than did haloperidol.

This effect was not evident in a retrospective case-control study of 27 patients with schizophrenia or schizoaffective disorder (Buckley et al. 1997). In these patients, a similar response between risperidone and typical antipsychotics was found, as measured by the use of restraints and seclusion. Another negative report found risperidone to be no different than typical neuroleptics in controlling aggressive behavior among a group of 20 forensic patients with chronic schizophrenia (Beck et al. 1997).

Methodological problems abound in studies of atypical antipsychotics in the treatment of aggressive behavior (Volavka and Citrome 1999), and thus interpretation of the literature is difficult.

Quetiapine. Quetiapine may also preferentially reduce hostility and aggression in patients with acute schizophrenia. From the data gathered on 351 patients in a 6-week placebo-controlled, double-blind, randomized efficacy-and-safety Phase III clinical trial, quetiapine was compared with haloperidol on measures of aggression and hostility assessed with the BPRS (Cantillon and Goldstein 1998). Quetiapine and haloperidol were both superior to placebo in reducing positive symptoms, but only quetiapine was superior to placebo on the measures of aggression and hostility.

Beta-Blockers

Beta-adrenergic blockers, in particular propranolol, have been used in the treatment of aggressive behavior in patients with brain injury (Yudofsky et al. 1981, 1984), but its use in patients with schizophrenia has not been as well examined (Volavka 1988, 1995). Propranolol has been used as an adjunctive treatment for schizophrenia, in which a reduction in symptoms, including aggression, was found (Sheppard 1979). A chart review of chronically assaultive schizophrenia patients who were receiving nadolol or propranolol revealed a 70% decrease in actual assaults for four of the seven patients (Sorgi et al. 1986). A double-blind, placebo-controlled study of adjunctive nadolol (40–120 mg/day) in 41 patients, 29 of whom were diagnosed with schizophrenia, found a decline in the frequency of aggression relative to control subjects (Ratey et al. 1992). In a preliminary report of a double-blind, placebo-controlled study of adjunctive nadolol (80–120 mg/day) in 30 violent inpatients, 23 of whom were diagnosed with schizophrenia, a trend was found demonstrating lower hostility for the active-treatment group (Alpert et al. 1990). A decrease in extrapyramidal symptoms was also noted, leading to the conclusion that antiaggression and anti-akathisia effects were associated; however, in the investigators' final report on 34 acutely aggressive male schizophrenia patients (Allan et al. 1996), this association was not maintained. Nadolol appeared to induce a more rapid decrease in overall psychiatric symptoms independently of any effect on extrapyramidal side effects.

Mood Stabilizers

Mood stabilizers such as lithium, valproate, and carbamazepine are used as adjuncts to neuroleptic treatment for patients with schizophrenia. In particular, valproate, in its two formulations valproic acid and divalproex sodium, is commonly used in the treatment of patients with schizophrenia. In 1996, 28.3% of 5,973 patients hospitalized with schizophrenia in state hospitals in New York received valproate (Citrome 1998).

In contrast to the literature on the use of valproate in the treatment of bipolar and schizoaffective disorders, very little is available on its use in the treatment of schizophrenia (McElroy et al. 1989; Wassef et al. 1999). Clinical lore suggests that valproate can be used to manage aggressivity, and this has been described in several case reports. Four patients with treatment-resistant schizophrenia were given valproate in addition to their neuroleptic medication, with a resulting reduction in both positive symptoms (as measured by the BPRS) and hostile/disruptive behavior (Morinigo et al. 1989). Two patients with schizophrenia and one with schizoaffective disorder were given valproate in addition to neuroleptics in an effort to control severe neuroleptic-resistant psychotic symptoms, with good results (Wassef et al. 1989). A comparison of valproate and carbamazepine in hospitalized patients (diagnosis not reported) revealed a decrease in the number of hours spent in mechanical restraints for both groups, with valproate being more effective than carbamazepine (Alam et al. 1995).

Given the widespread use of valproate, we are in need of more definitive studies on its effectiveness as an adjunctive agent for the control of agitation in psychotic patients. Double-blind, placebo-controlled studies are needed to prove the efficacy of valproate for this indication. As with both lithium and carbamazepine, an empirical trial of valproate may be considered for an individual patient, but chronic use, without demonstrable benefit, only exposes the patient to the possibility of side effects.

Both lithium and carbamazepine have also been prescribed in the treatment of patients with schizophrenia, although not as extensively as valproate at present. In 1993, at one state hospital (Citrome 1995; L. Citrome, unpublished data, 1993), approximately 15% of the patients diagnosed with schizophrenia were receiving at least one mood stabilizer (usually carbamazepine), and 86% of the time the indication for its (their) use was poor impulse control or assaultive/aggressive behavior. Monotherapy with carbamazepine or valproic acid resulted in statistically fewer adverse effects than with lithium or with combination therapy. The measure of effectiveness in reducing aggressivity was hampered by the reliance on data contained in the medical record, but the overall impression was that there was a tangible clinical benefit.

Studies looking at the usefulness of carbamazepine in the control of aggressive behavior in patients with schizophrenia are few in number (Volavka 1995). Eight women diagnosed with schizophrenia (some with EEG abnormalities) and exhibiting violent behavior were given carbamazepine in addition to their regular neuroleptic medication, with good results (Hakola and Laulumaa 1982). In a retrospective look at violent patients with and without abnormalities on the EEG, most of whom were diagnosed with schizophrenia, significant reductions in aggressivity were noted with carbamazepine, regardless of the patient's EEG status (Luchins 1984). A multifacility double-blind study compared the effect of a 4-week trial of carbamazepine with that of placebo as an adjunct to standard neuroleptic treatment (Okuma et al. 1989). Of the 162 patients, 78% had a DSM-III diagnosis of schizophrenia (the remainder were diagnosed with schizoaffective disorder), and all these patients exhibited excited states or aggressive/violent behavior that responded unsatisfactorily to neuroleptic treatment. There was no statistically significant difference in response among the patients with schizophrenia receiving either adjunctive carbamazepine or placebo, but a trend toward moderate improvement with carbamazepine was noted ($P < 0.10$). A 15-week double-blind, randomized, within-patient crossover study assessed the efficacy of adjunctive carbamazepine in 13 nonepileptic chronic inpatients with EEG temporal lobe abnormalities (Neppe 1983, 1988). Nine of the patients were diagnosed with schizophrenia, and 7 of the 13 completed the study. Overt aggression was rated as 2 times as severe and 1.5 times as common when the patients were receiving placebo as when they were receiving carbamazepine. Response was not correlated with EEG deterioration or improvement.

With rare exceptions, the published studies of carbamazepine and aggressivity were not blinded and did not control for placebo effect. In addition, plasma levels of concomitant neuroleptics were not measured, leaving open the possibility for undetected pharmacokinetic interactions. Despite these limitations, carbamazepine appears to be a useful adjunct to neuroleptic therapy (Simhandl and Meszaros 1992) and may lower aggression in a broad spectrum of disorders, including schizophrenia (Young and Hillbrand 1994).

The effectiveness of lithium therapy in patients with schizophrenia is not established. Prior studies that demonstrated benefits are plagued with methodological problems such as small sample size and lack of strict diagnostic criteria (Atre-Vaidya and Taylor 1989). Active affective symptoms, previous affective episodes, and a family history of affective disorder may predict a favorable response to lithium (Atre-Vaidya and Taylor 1989) but also provide clues that the diagnosis may be something other than schizophrenia (Citrome 1989). A double-blind, placebo-controlled, parallel-design clinical trial involving seriously ill state hospital patients with schizophrenia who had not responded to prior trials of typical neuroleptics demonstrated no advantage of lithium combined with haloperidol over haloperidol alone (Wilson 1993). When lithium was added to neuroleptics for patients with treatment-resistant schizophrenia who were classified as "dangerous, violent or criminal," no benefits were seen after 4 weeks of adjunctive lithium (Collins et al. 1991). Another group found that lithium was useful as a single agent in ameliorating psychosis in three schizophrenia patients who exhibited marked akathisia and accompanying agitation, restlessness, and irritability when they were receiving standard neuroleptics (Shalev et al. 1987). For some schizophrenia patients, the impact of lithium on core psychotic symptoms (hallucinations, delusions, formal thought disorder) may be evident after the first 7 days (Zemlan et al. 1984). There are case reports of patients with paranoid schizophrenia with aggressive or disorderly behaviors who have responded to the addition of lithium to their neuroleptic treatment, then deteriorated after the lithium was discontinued, but subsequently improved when it was reinstituted (Prakash 1985).

Clonazepam

Clonazepam, a high-potency benzodiazepine, was reported to be useful as an antiaggressive agent in a case report of a schizophrenia patient with a seizure disorder (Keats and Mukherjee 1988). In this particular case, both phenytoin and carbamazepine were ineffective. The patient did best on a combination of haloperidol and clonazepam. This result is in contrast to a double-blind, placebo-controlled trial of adjunctive clonazepam in 13 schizophrenia patients who were receiving neuroleptics (Karson et al. 1982). In that study, no additional therapeutic benefit was observed, and, in fact, four patients demonstrated violent behavior during the course of clonazepam treatment.

Antidepressants

The current interest in the role of certain antidepressants in aggression is based on the crucial role of serotonergic regulation of impulsive aggression against self and others. Now that antidepressants with specific effects on serotonin (5-HT) receptors have become available, a number of reports have emerged. In a retrospective, uncontrolled study, adjunctive fluoxetine, a selective serotonin reuptake inhibitor (SSRI), was given to five patients with chronic schizophrenia, with a decrease in violent incidents observed in four of the patients (Goldman and Janecek 1990).

Citalopram, an SSRI that is now available in the United States, was tested for antiaggressive effects in 15 chronically violent hospitalized schizophrenia patients (Vartiainen et al. 1995). This double-blind, placebo-controlled, crossover study lasted 48 weeks (24 weeks on active citalopram, 24 weeks on citalopram placebo). The trial medication was added to the concurrent neuroleptic treatment. The number of aggressive incidents decreased during the active citalopram treatment.

In a case report, the addition of fluvoxamine (another SSRI) to risperidone was reported to be effective in managing aggression in patients with schizophrenia (Silver and Kushnir 1998).

Outpatient Management

Outpatient commitment may be an option in some states (Torrey and Kaplan 1995) and may improve compliance with treatment. This improved compliance in turn would decrease the frequency of relapse due to noncompliance. For patients with a known history of violent and aggressive behaviors when not taking medication, outpatient commitment may be a viable alternative to continued hospitalization.

Summary

Violent or threatening behavior is a frequent reason for admission to a psychiatric inpatient facility, and such behavior may continue after the admission. For patients with schizophrenia, the association between preadmission threats and postadmission violence is impressive. Patients who have been chronically hospitalized may also be aggressive. The distinction between transient and recidivistic assaultiveness is important; a small group of recidivistic patients may cause the majority of violent incidents.

Patients with schizophrenia and aggressive behavior must first be assessed for the possibility of comorbid conditions. The presence of a comorbid substance use disorder greatly increases the risk of aggressive behavior. Medical conditions, including acute withdrawal from alcohol or sedatives, need to be ruled out. A risk assessment that includes past history and access to weapons is vital. Beyond the acute management of an aggressive episode, long-term management will depend on the pattern of violence (i.e., whether it is transient or persistent).

Short-term sedation with lorazepam is a safe and effective choice for the acute episode. Use of neuroleptics may lead to side effects such as akathisia, which may in turn precipitate further agitation. The advent of intramuscular preparations of atypical antipsychotics may obviate this problem. Concomitant use of restraints may be necessary to prevent injury to self or others. An interdisciplinary approach requires staff training in the management of crisis situations.

Longer-term management may include the use of a specialized hospital unit, if available. Preventive aggression devices may be helpful. Pharmacotherapy remains the mainstay of treatment. Lorazepam for long-term daily use is not recommended because of problems associated with tolerance, dependence, and withdrawal. Clozapine appears to be more effective than typical neuroleptics in reducing aggressivity in patients with schizophrenia and stands out among the other atypical antipsychotics in this regard. Beta-blockers, well studied in the treatment of aggressive behavior in patients with brain injury, also may be helpful as an adjunct to neuroleptics for aggression and schizophrenia. Carbamazepine and valproate are also used with neuroleptics to decrease the intensity and frequency of agitation and poor impulse control, but they have not been extensively studied under double-blind, placebo-controlled conditions in this population. The efficacy of lithium has not been established for patients with schizophrenia, but there are case reports that document its utility in specific situations.

Outpatient commitment might enable some chronically hospitalized patients with schizophrenia and aggression to live in the community. With the downsizing and elimination of state psychiatric hospitals, this alternative to hospitalization appears critical to protect both the patient and the public.

References

Alam MY, Klass DB, Luchins DJ, et al: Effectiveness of divalproex sodium, valproic acid and carbamazepine in aggression. Poster presented at the 35th annual meeting of the New Clinical Drug Evaluation Unit, Boca Raton, FL, June 1995

Allan E, Alpert M, Sison C, et al: Adjunctive nadolol in the treatment of acutely aggressive schizophrenic patients. J Clin Psychiatry 57:455–459, 1996

Alpert M, Allan ER, Citrome L, et al: A double-blind, placebo-controlled study of adjunctive nadolol in the management of violent psychiatric patients. Psychopharmacol Bull 26:367–371, 1990

American Psychiatric Association: Diagnostic and Statistical Manual of Mental Disorders, 4th Edition, Text Revision. Washington, DC, American Psychiatric Association, 2000

Apter A, Van Praag HM, Plutchik R, et al: Interrelationships among anxiety, aggression, impulsivity, and mood: a serotonergically linked cluster? Psychiatry Res 32:191–199, 1990

Atre-Vaidya N, Taylor MA: Effectiveness of lithium in schizophrenia: do we really have an answer? J Clin Psychiatry 50:170–173, 1989

Beaudoin MN, Hodgins S, Lavoie F: Homicide, schizophrenia and substance abuse or dependency. Can J Psychiatry 38:541–546, 1993

Beck NC, Greenfield SR, Gotham H, et al: Risperidone in the management of violent, treatment-resistant schizophrenics hospitalized in a maximum security forensic facility. J Am Acad Psychiatry Law 25:461–468, 1997

Binder RL, McNiel DE: Effects of diagnosis and context on dangerousness. Am J Psychiatry 145:728–732, 1988

Blomhoff S, Seim S, Friis S: Can prediction of violence among psychiatric inpatients be improved? Hospital and Community Psychiatry 41:771–775, 1990

Bond A, Lader M: Benzodiazepines and aggression, in Psychopharmacology of Aggression, Edited by Sandler M. New York, Raven, 1979, pp 173–182

Boxer PA: Assessment of potential violence in the paranoid worker. Journal of Occupational Medicine 35:127–131, 1993

Brailsford DS, Stevenson J: Factors related to violent and unpredictable behavior in psychiatric hospitals. Nursing Times 69 (suppl, January 18):9–11, 1973

Brown GL, Goodwin FK, Ballenger JC, et al: Aggression in humans correlates with cerebrospinal fluid amine metabolites. Psychiatry Res 1:131–139, 1979

Buchanan A: The investigation of acting on delusions as a tool for risk assessment in the mentally disordered. Br J Psychiatry 170 (suppl 32):12–16, 1997

Buckley P, Bartell J, Donenwirth MA, et al: Violence and schizophrenia: clozapine as a specific antiaggressive agent. Bull Am Acad Psychiatry Law 23:607–611, 1995

Buckley PF, Ibrahim ZY, Singer B, et al: Aggression and schizophrenia: efficacy of risperidone. J Am Psychiatry Law 25:173–181, 1997

Buss AH, Durkee A: An inventory for assessing different kinds of hostility. Journal of Consulting Psychology 21:343–349, 1957

Calcedo-Barba AL, Calcedo-Ordonez A: Violence and paranoid schizophrenia. Int J Law Psychiatry 17:253–263, 1994

Cantillon M, Goldstein JM: Quetiapine fumarate reduces aggression and hostility in patients with schizophrenia (NR444), in 1998 New Research Program and Abstracts, American Psychiatric Association 151st Annual Meeting, Toronto, Ontario, Canada, May 30–June 4, 1998. Washington, DC, American Psychiatric Association, 1998

Cheung P, Schweitzer I, Crowley K, et al: Violence in schizophrenia: role of hallucinations and delusions. Schizophr Res 26:181–190, 1997

Chiles JA, Davidson P, McBride D: Effects of clozapine on use of seclusion and restraint at a state hospital. Hospital and Community Psychiatry 45:269–271, 1994

Citrome L: Differential diagnosis of psychosis. Postgrad Med 85:273–280, 1989

Citrome L: Use of lithium, carbamazepine, and valproic acid in a state-operated psychiatric hospital. Journal of Pharmacy Technology 11:55–59, 1995

Citrome L: New antipsychotic medications: what advantages do they offer? Postgrad Med 101:207–214, 1997

Citrome L: Valproate: extent of use within the inpatient population of the New York State Office of Mental Health psychiatric hospital system. Psychiatr Q 69:283–300, 1998

Citrome L, Green L: The dangerous agitated patient: what to do right now. Postgrad Med 87:231–236, 1990

Citrome L, Green L, Fost R: Clinical and administrative consequences of a reduced census on a psychiatric intensive care unit. Psychiatr Q 66:209–217, 1995

Clinton JE, Sterner S, Stelmachers Z, et al: Haloperidol for sedation of disruptive emergency patients. Ann Emerg Med 16:319–322, 1987

Cobb CD, Anderson CB, Seidel DR: Possible interaction between clozapine and lorazepam (letter). Am J Psychiatry 148:1606–1607, 1991

Coccaro EF, Siever LJ, Klar HM, et al: Serotonergic studies in patients with affective and personality disorders. Arch Gen Psychiatry 46:587–599, 1989

Collins PJ, Larkin EP, Shubsachs APW: Lithium carbonate in chronic schizophrenia—a brief trial of lithium carbonate added to neuroleptics for treatment of resistant schizophrenic patients. Acta Psychiatr Scand 84:150–154, 1991

Convit A, Jaeger J, Lin SP, et al: Predicting assaultiveness in psychiatric inpatients: a pilot study. Hospital and Community Psychiatry 39:429–434, 1988

Convit A, Isay D, Otis D, et al: Characteristics of repeatedly assaultive psychiatric inpatients. Hospital and Community Psychiatry 41:1112–1115, 1990

Convit A, Czobor P, Volavka J: Lateralized abnormality in the EEG of persistently violent psychiatric inpatients. Biol Psychiatry 30:363–370, 1991

Convit A, Volavka J, Czobor P, et al: Effect of subtle neurological dysfunction on response to haloperidol treatment in schizophrenia. Am J Psychiatry 151:49–56, 1994

Convit A, Douyon R, Yates K, et al: Fronto-temporal abnormalities in violence, in Aggression and Violence: Genetic, Neurobiological and Biosocial Perspectives. Edited by Stoff D, Cairns R. Hillside, NJ, Erlbaum, 1996, pp 169–194

Cuffel BJ: Prevalence estimates of substance abuse in schizophrenia and their correlates. J Nerv Ment Dis 180:589–592, 1992

Cuffel BJ, Shumway M, Chouljian TL, et al: A longitudinal study of substance abuse and community violence in schizophrenia. J Nerv Ment Dis 182:704–708, 1994

Czobor P, Volavka J: Violence in the mentally ill: questions remain (letter). Arch Gen Psychiatry 56:193–194, 1999

Czobor P, Volavka J, Meibach RC: Effect of risperidone on hostility in schizophrenia. J Clin Psychopharmacol 15:243–249, 1995

Dietch JT, Jennings RK: Aggressive dyscontrol in patients treated with benzodiazepines. J Clin Psychiatry 49:184–188, 1988

Donlon PT, Hopkin J, Tupin J: Overview: efficacy and safety of the rapid neuroleptization method with injectable haloperidol. Am J Psychiatry 136:273–278, 1979

Ebrahim GM, Gibler B, Gacono CB, et al: Patient response to clozapine in a forensic psychiatric hospital. Hospital and Community Psychiatry 45:271–273, 1994

Eichelman BS, Hartwig AC (eds): Patient Violence and the Clinician. Washington, DC, American Psychiatric Press, 1995

Eronen M, Hakola P, Tiihonen J: Mental disorders and homicidal behavior in Finland. Arch Gen Psychiatry 53:497–501, 1996

Fisher WA: Restraint and seclusion: a review of the literature. Am J Psychiatry 151:1584–1591, 1994

Fottrell E: A study of violent behavior among patients in psychiatric hospitals. Br J Psychiatry 136:216–221, 1980

Friedman LJ, Tabb SE, Worthington JJ, et al: Clozapine—a novel antipsychotic agent (letter). N Engl J Med 325:518, 1991

Geller MP: Sociopathic adaptations in psychotic patients. Hospital and Community Psychiatry 31:108–112, 1980

Gertz B: Training for prevention of assaultive behavior in a psychiatric setting. Hospital and Community Psychiatry 31:628–630, 1980

Gibson RW: On the therapeutic handling of aggression in schizophrenia. Am J Orthopsychiatry 37:926–931, 1967

Glazer WM, Dickson RA: Clozapine reduces violence and persistent aggression in schizophrenia. J Clin Psychiatry 59 (no 3, suppl):8–14, 1998

Goldman MB, Janecek HM: Adjunctive fluoxetine improves global function in chronic schizophrenia. J Neuropsychiatry Clin Neurosci 2:429–431, 1990

Goldney R, Bowes J, Spence N, et al: The psychiatric intensive care unit. Br J Psychiatry 146:50–54, 1985

Greenblatt DJ, Shader RI, Franke K, et al: Pharmacokinetics and bioavailability of intravenous, intramuscular, and oral lorazepam in humans. J Pharm Sci 68:57–63, 1979

Greenblatt DJ, Divoll M, Harmatz JS, et al: Pharmacokinetic comparison of sublingual lorazepam with intravenous, intramuscular, and oral lorazepam. J Pharm Sci 71:248–252, 1982

Hakola HP, Laulumaa VA: Carbamazepine in treatment of violent schizophrenics (letter). Lancet 1:1358, 1982

Hamstra B: Neurobiological substrates of violence: an overview for forensic clinicians. Journal of Psychiatry and Law Fall–Winter 1986, pp 349–374

Hodgins S: Mental disorder, intellectual deficiency, and crime: evidence from a birth cohort. Arch Gen Psychiatry 49:476–483, 1992

Hodgins S, Mednick SA, Brennan PA, et al: Mental disorder and crime: evidence from a Danish birth cohort. Arch Gen Psychiatry 53:489–496, 1996

Humphreys MS, Johnstone EC, MacMillan JF, et al: Dangerous behavior preceding first admission for schizophrenia. Br J Psychiatry 161:501–505, 1992

Junginger J: Command hallucinations and the prediction of dangerousness. Psychiatr Serv 46:911–914, 1995

Junginger J, Parks-Levy J, McGuire L: Delusions and symptom-consistent violence. Psychiatr Serv 49:218–220, 1998

Kanofsky JD, Lindenmayer JP: Relapse in a clozapine responder following lorazepam withdrawal (letter). Am J Psychiatry 150:348–349, 1993 [Published erratum Am J Psychiatry 150:685, 1993]

Kapur S, Remington G: Serotonin-dopamine interaction and its relevance to schizophrenia. Am J Psychiatry 153:466–476, 1996

Karson C, Bigelow LB: Violent behavior in schizophrenic inpatients. J Nerv Ment Dis 175:161–164, 1987

Karson CN, Weinberger DR, Bigelow L, et al: Clonazepam treatment of chronic schizophrenia: negative results in a double-blind, placebo-controlled trial. Am J Psychiatry 139:1627–1628, 1982

Keats MM, Mukherjee S: Antiaggressive effect of adjunctive clonazepam in schizophrenia associated with seizure disorder. J Clin Psychiatry 49:117–118, 1988

Keckich WA: Neuroleptics. Violence as a manifestation of akathisia. JAMA 240:2185, 1978

Klimke A, Klieser E: Sudden death after intravenous application of lorazepam in a patient treated with clozapine (letter). Am J Psychiatry 151:780, 1994

Koczapski AB, Ledwidge B, Paredes J, et al: Multisubstance intoxication among schizophrenic inpatients: reply to Hyde. Schizophr Bull 16:373–375, 1990

Koo JYM, Chien CP: Coma following ECT and intravenous droperidol: case report. J Clin Psychiatry 47:94–95, 1986

Krakowski M, Czobor P: Violence in psychiatric patients: the role of psychosis, frontal lobe impairment, and ward turmoil. Compr Psychiatry 38:230–236, 1997

Krakowski M, Volavka J, Brizer D: Psychopathology and violence: a review of the literature. Compr Psychiatry 27:131–148, 1986

Krakowski M, Convit A, Volavka J: Patterns of inpatient assaultiveness: effect of neurological impairment and deviant family environment on response to treatment. Neuropsychiatry Neuropsychol Behav Neurol 1:21–29, 1988

Krakowski M, Convit A, Jaeger J, et al: Inpatient violence: trait and state. J Psychiatr Res 23:57–64, 1989a

Krakowski M, Convit A, Jaeger J, et al: Neurological impairment in violent schizophrenic inpatients. Am J Psychiatry 146:849–853, 1989b

Krakowski MI, Kunz M, Czobor P, et al: Long-term high-dose neuroleptic treatment: who gets it and why? Hospital and Community Psychiatry 44:640–644, 1993

Kunz M, Sikora J, Krakowski M, et al: Serotonin in violent patients with schizophrenia. Psychiatry Res 59:161–163, 1995

Lalemand K: Advanced NAPPI Training for Rockland Psychiatric Center, Non-Abusive Psychological and Physical Intervention, Participant Manual. Auburn, ME, Non-Abusive Psychological and Physical Intervention, 1998

Lane FE: Utilizing physician empathy with violent patients. Am J Psychother 40:448–456, 1986

Lehmann LS, Padilla M, Clark S, et al: Training personnel in the prevention and management of violent behavior. Hospital and Community Psychiatry 34:40–43, 1983

Lindqvist P, Allebeck P: Schizophrenia and assaultive behaviour: the role of alcohol and drug abuse. Acta Psychiatr Scand 82:191–195, 1990

Link BG, Stueve A: Psychotic symptoms and the violent/illegal behavior of mental patients compared to community controls, in Violence and Mental Disorder: Developments in Risk Assessment. Edited by Monahan J, Steadman HJ. Chicago, IL, University of Chicago Press, 1994, pp 137–159

Link BG, Cullen FT, Andrews H: The violent and illegal behavior of mental patients reconsidered. American Sociological Review 57:275–292, 1992

Linnoila M, Virkkunen M, Scheinin M, et al: Low cerebrospinal fluid 5-hydroxyindole acetic acid concentration differentiates impulsive from non-impulsive violent behavior. Life Sci 33:2609–2614, 1983

Lion JR, Synder W, Merrill GL: Underreporting of assaults on staff in a state hospital. Hospital and Community Psychiatry 32:497–498, 1981

Lothstein LM, Jones P: Discriminating violent individuals by means of various psychological tests. J Pers Assess 42:237–243, 1978

Luchins DJ: Carbamazepine in violent non-epileptic schizophrenics. Psychopharmacol Bull 20:569–571, 1984

Maguire K, Pastore AL (eds): Sourcebook of Criminal Justice Statistics 1996. Washington, DC, U.S. Department of Justice, Bureau of Justice Statistics, 1997 [http://www.albany.edu/sourcebook]

Maier GJ: The impact of clozapine on 25 forensic patients. Bull Am Acad Psychiatry Law 20:297–307, 1992

Maier GJ, Stava LJ, Morrow BR, et al: A model for understanding and managing cycles of aggression among psychiatric inpatients. Hospital and Community Psychiatry 38:520–524, 1987

Mallya AR, Roos PD, Roebuck-Colgan K: Restraint, seclusion, and clozapine. J Clin Psychiatry 53:395–397, 1992

Marder SR, Meibach RC: Risperidone in the treatment of schizophrenia. Am J Psychiatry 151:825–835, 1994

Martell DA: Estimating the prevalence of organic brain dysfunction in maximum-security forensic psychiatric patients. J Forensic Sci 37:878–893, 1992

McElroy SL, Keck PE, Pope HG, et al: Valproate in psychiatric disorders: literature review and clinical guidelines. J Clin Psychiatry 50 (no 3, suppl):23–29, 1989

McNiel DE: Hallucinations and violence, in Violence and Mental Disorder: Developments in Risk Assessment. Edited by Monahan J, Steadman HJ. Chicago, IL, University of Chicago Press, 1994, pp 183–202

McNiel DE, Binder RL: Relationship between preadmission threats and later violent behavior by acute psychiatric inpatients. Hospital and Community Psychiatry 40:605–608, 1989

McNiel DE, Binder RL: Correlates of accuracy in the assessment of psychiatric inpatients' risk of violence. Am J Psychiatry 152:901–906, 1995

Mendez MF, Doss RC, Taylor JL: Interictal violence in epilepsy. J Nerv Ment Dis 181:566–569, 1993

Monahan J: Limiting therapist exposure to Tarasoff liability: guidelines for risk containment. Am Psychol 48:242–250, 1993

Morinigo A, Martin J, Gonzalez S, et al: Treatment of resistant schizophrenia with valproate and neuroleptic drugs. Hillside J Clin Psychiatry 11:199–207, 1989

Mueser KT, Drake RE, Ackerson TH, et al: Antisocial personality disorder, conduct disorder, and substance abuse in schizophrenia. J Abnorm Psychol 106:473–477, 1997

Musisi SM, Wasylenki DA, Rapp MS: A psychiatric intensive care unit in a psychiatric hospital. Can J Psychiatry 34:200–204, 1989

Neborsky R, Janowsky D, Munson E, et al: Rapid treatment of acute psychotic symptoms with high- and low-dose haloperidol. Arch Gen Psychiatry 38:195–199, 1981

Neppe VM: Carbamazepine as adjunctive treatment in nonepileptic chronic inpatients with EEG temporal lobe abnormalities. J Clin Psychiatry 44:326–331, 1983

Neppe VM: Carbamazepine in nonresponsive psychosis. J Clin Psychiatry 49 (no 4, suppl):22–28, 1988

Newhill CE, Mulvey EP, Lidz CW: Characteristics of violence in the community by female patients seen in a psychiatric emergency service. Psychiatr Serv 46:785–789, 1995

Okuma T, Yamashita I, Takahashi R, et al: A double-blind study of adjunctive carbamazepine versus placebo on excited states of schizophrenic and schizoaffective disorders. Acta Psychiatr Scand 80:250–259, 1989

Owen C, Tarantello C, Jones M, et al: Repetitively violent patients in psychiatric units. Psychiatr Serv 49:1458–1461, 1998a

Owen C, Tarantello C, Jones M, et al: Violence and aggression in psychiatric units. Psychiatr Serv 49:1452–1457, 1998b

Palmstierna T, Huitfeldt B, Wistedt B: The relationship of crowding and aggressive behavior on a psychiatric intensive care unit. Hospital and Community Psychiatry 42:1237–1240, 1991

Plutchik R, Van Praag H: Psychosocial correlates of suicide and violence risk, in Violence and Suicidality: Perspectives in Clinical and Psychobiological Research. Edited by Van Praag HM, Plutchik R, Apter A. New York, Brunner/Mazel, 1990, pp 37–65

Plutchik R, Van Praag HM, Conte HR: Correlates of suicide and violence risk, III: a two-stage model of countervailing forces. Psychiatry Res 28:215–225, 1989

Prakash R: Lithium-responsive schizophrenia: case reports. J Clin Psychiatry 46:141–142, 1985

Rasanen P, Tiihonen J, Isohanni M, et al: Schizophrenia, alcohol abuse, and violent behavior: a 26-year followup study of an unselected birth cohort. Schizophr Bull 24:437–441, 1998

Ratey JJ, Sorgi P, O'Driscoll GA, et al: Nadolol to treat aggression and psychiatric symptomatology in chronic psychiatric inpatients: a double-blind, placebo-controlled study. J Clin Psychiatry 53:41–46, 1992

Ratey JJ, Leveroni C, Kilmer D, et al: The effects of clozapine on severely aggressive psychiatric inpatients in a state hospital. J Clin Psychiatry 54:219–223, 1993

Reeves KR, Swift RH, Harrigan EP: Intramuscular ziprasidone 20 mg in acute agitation (NR495), in 1998 New Research Program and Abstracts, American Psychiatric Association 151st Annual Meeting, Toronto, Ontario, Canada, May 30–June 4, 1998. Washington, DC, American Psychiatric Association, 1998a

Reeves KR, Swift RH, Harrigan EP: Ziprasidone intramuscular 10 mg and 20 mg in acute agitation (NR494), in 1998 New Research Program and Abstracts, American Psychiatric Association 151st Annual Meeting, Toronto, Ontario, Canada, May 30–June 4, 1998. Washington, DC, American Psychiatric Association, 1998b

Regier DA, Farmer ME, Rae DS, et al: Comorbidity of mental disorders with alcohol and other drug abuse: results from the Epidemiologic Catchment Area (ECA) Study. JAMA 264:2511–2518, 1990

Robins LN: Deviant Children Grown Up: A Sociological and Psychiatric Study of Sociopathic Personality. Baltimore, MD, Williams & Wilkins, 1966

Robins LN, Tipp J, Przybeck T: Antisocial personality, in Psychiatric Disorders in America: The Epidemiologic Catchment Area Study. Edited by Robins LN, Regier DA. New York, Free Press, 1991, pp 258–290

Rogers R, Seman W: Murder and criminal responsibility: an examination of MMPI profiles. Behav Sci Law 1:90–95, 1983

Rogers R, Nussbaum D, Gillis R: Command hallucinations and criminality: a clinical quandary. Bull Am Acad Psychiatry Law 16:251–258, 1988

Roy A, Linnoila M: Suicidal behavior, impulsiveness and serotonin. Acta Psychiatr Scand 78:529–535, 1988

Salzman C: Use of benzodiazepines to control disruptive behavior in inpatients. J Clin Psychiatry 49 (no 12, suppl):13–15, 1988

Schatzberg AF, Cole JO: Manual of Clinical Psychopharmacology, 2nd Edition. Washington, DC, American Psychiatric Press, 1991, p 99

Shalev A, Hermesh H, Munitz H: Severe akathisia causing neuroleptic failure: an indication for lithium therapy in schizophrenia? Acta Psychiatr Scand 76:715–718, 1987

Sheppard GP: High-dose propranolol in schizophrenia. Br J Psychiatry 134:470–476, 1979

Shore D, Filson CR, Johnson WE: Violent crime arrests and paranoid schizophrenia: the White House case studies. Schizophr Bull 14:279–281, 1988

Silver H, Kushnir M: Treatment of aggression in schizophrenia (letter). Am J Psychiatry 155:1298, 1998

Silver JM, Yudofsky SC: The Overt Aggression Scale: overview and guiding principles. J Neuropsychiatry Clin Neurosci 3(suppl):S22–S29, 1991

Simhandl C, Meszaros K: The use of carbamazepine in the treatment of schizophrenic and schizoaffective psychoses: a review. J Psychiatr Neurosci 17:1–14, 1992

Siris SG: Three cases of akathisia and "acting out." J Clin Psychiatry 46:395–397, 1985

Smith J, Hucker S: Schizophrenia and substance abuse. Br J Psychiatry 165:13–21, 1994

Sorgi PJ, Ratey JJ, Polakoff S: Beta-adrenergic blockers for the control of aggressive behaviors in patients with chronic schizophrenia. Am J Psychiatry 143:775–776, 1986

Spellacy F: Neuropsychological discrimination between violent and non-violent men. J Clin Psychol 34:49–52, 1978

Spivak B, Mester R, Wittenberg N, et al: Reduction of aggressiveness and impulsiveness during clozapine treatment in chronic neuroleptic-resistant schizophrenic patients. Clin Neuropharmacol 20:442–446, 1997

Steadman HJ, Mulvey EP, Monahan J, et al: Violence by people discharged from acute psychiatric inpatient facilities and others in the same neighborhoods. Arch Gen Psychiatry 55:393–401, 1998

Swanson JW: Mental disorder, substance abuse, and community violence: an epidemiological approach, in Violence and Mental Disorder: Developments in Risk Assessment. Edited by Monahan J, Steadman HJ. Chicago, IL, University of Chicago Press, 1994, pp 101–136

Swartz MS, Swanson JW, Hiday VA, et al: Violence and severe mental illness: the effects of substance abuse and nonadherence to medication. Am J Psychiatry 155:226–231, 1998

Swift RH, Harrigan EP, van Kammen DP: A comparison of intramuscular ziprasidone with intramuscular haloperidol (NR465), in 1998 New Research Program and Abstracts, American Psychiatric Association 151st Annual Meeting, Toronto, Ontario, Canada, May 30–June 4, 1998. Washington, DC, American Psychiatric Association, 1998

Tanke ED, Yesavage JA: Characteristics of assaultive patients who do and do not provide visible cues of potential violence. Am J Psychiatry 142:1409–1413, 1985

Tardiff K: The current state of psychiatry in the treatment of violent patients. Arch Gen Psychiatry 49:493–499, 1992

Tardiff K, Sweillam A: Assaultive behavior among chronic inpatients. Am J Psychiatry 139:212–215, 1982

Taylor PJ: Motives for offending among violent and psychotic men. Br J Psychiatry 147:491–498, 1985

Thackrey M: Therapeutics for Aggression: Psychological/Physical Crisis Intervention. New York, Human Sciences Press, 1987

Thomas H, Schwartz E, Petrilli R: Droperidol versus haloperidol for chemical restraint of agitated and combative patients. Ann Emerg Med 21:407–413, 1992

Torrey EF, Kaplan RJ: A national survey on the use of outpatient commitment. Psychiatr Serv 46:778–784, 1995

Travin S, Protter B: Mad or bad? Some clinical considerations in the misdiagnosis of schizophrenia as antisocial personality disorder. Am J Psychiatry 139:1335–1338, 1982

Tupin JP: The violent patient: a strategy for management and diagnosis. Hospital and Community Psychiatry 34:37–40, 1983

Van Rybroek GJ, Kuhlman TL, Maier GJ, et al: Preventive aggression devices (PADS): ambulatory restraints as an alternative to seclusion. J Clin Psychiatry 48:401–405, 1987

Vartiainen H, Tiihonen J, Putkonen A, et al: Citalopram, a selective serotonin reuptake inhibitor, in the treatment of aggression in schizophrenia. Acta Psychiatr Scand 91:348–351, 1995

Victor M: Treatment of alcohol intoxication and the withdrawal syndrome. Psychosom Med 28 (no 4, pt 2):636–650, 1966

Virkkunen M: Observations on violence in schizophrenia. Acta Psychiatr Scand 50:145–151, 1974

Virkkunen M, Linnoila M: Serotonin in early onset, male alcoholics with violent behaviour. Ann Med 22:327–331, 1990

Virkkunen M, De Jong J, Bartko J, et al: Psychobiological concomitants of history of suicide attempts among violent offenders and impulsive fire setters. Arch Gen Psychiatry 46:604–606, 1989

Virkkunen M, Goldman D, Nielsen DA, et al: Low brain serotonin turnover rate (low CSF 5-HIAA) and impulsive violence. J Psychiatry Neurosci 20:271–275, 1995

Volavka J: Can aggressive behavior in humans be modified by beta blockers? Postgrad Med February 29 (special report), 1988, pp 163–168

Volavka J: Neurobiology of Violence. Washington, DC, American Psychiatric Press, 1995

Volavka J, Citrome L: Atypical antipsychotics in the treatment of the persistently aggressive psychotic patient: methodological concerns. Schizophr Res 35(suppl): S23–S33, 1999

Volavka J, Krakowski M: Schizophrenia and violence. Psychol Med 19:559–562, 1989

Volavka J, Martell D, Convit A: Psychobiology of the violent offender. J Forensic Sci 37:237–251, 1992

Volavka J, Zito JM, Vitrai J, et al: Clozapine effects on hostility and aggression in schizophrenia. J Clin Psychopharmacol 13:287–289, 1993

Volavka J, Laska E, Baker S, et al: History of violent behavior and schizophrenia in different cultures. Br J Psychiatry 171:9–14, 1997

Wallace C, Mullen P, Burgess P, et al: Serious criminal offending and mental disorder. Br J Psychiatry 172:477–484, 1998

Warneke L: A psychiatric intensive care unit in a general hospital setting. Can J Psychiatry 31:834–837, 1986

Wassef A, Watson D, Morrison P, et al: Neuroleptic-valproic acid combination in treatment of psychotic symptoms: a three-case report. J Clin Psychopharmacol 9:45–48, 1989

Wassef AA, Dott SG, Harris A, et al: Critical review of GABA-ergic drugs in the treatment of schizophrenia. J Clin Psychopharmacol 19:222–232, 1999

Weiger WA, Bear DM: An approach to the neurology of aggression. J Psychiatr Res 22:85–98, 1988

Weinberger DR, Berman KF, Zec RF: Physiologic dysfunction of dorsolateral prefrontal cortex in schizophrenia, I: regional cerebral blood flow evidence. Arch Gen Psychiatry 43:114–124, 1986

Wilson WH: Addition of lithium to haloperidol in non-affective, antipsychotic nonresponsive schizophrenia: a double blind, placebo controlled parallel design clinical trial. Psychopharmacology (Berl) 111:359–366, 1993

Wilson WH, Claussen AM: Eighteen-month outcome of clozapine treatment for 100 patients in a state psychiatric hospital. Psychiatr Serv 46:386–389, 1995

Yesavage JA: Inpatient violence and the schizophrenic patient: an inverse correlation between danger-related events and neuroleptic levels. Biol Psychiatry 17:1331–1337, 1982

Yesavage JA: Dangerous behavior by Vietnam veterans with schizophrenia. Am J Psychiatry 140:1180–1183, 1983a

Yesavage JA: Differential effects of Vietnam combat experiences vs. criminality on dangerous behavior by Vietnam veterans with schizophrenia. J Nerv Ment Dis 171:382–384, 1983b

Young JL, Hillbrand M: Carbamazepine lowers aggression: a review. Bull Am Acad Psychiatry Law 22:53–61, 1994

Yudofsky S, Williams D, Gorman J: Propranolol in the treatment of rage and violent behavior in patients with chronic brain syndrome. Am J Psychiatry 138:218–220, 1981

Yudofsky SC, Stevens L, Silver JM, et al: Propranolol in the treatment of rage and violent behavior associated with Korsakoff's psychosis. Am J Psychiatry 141:114–115, 1984

Yudofsky SC, Silver JM, Jackson W, et al: The Overt Aggression Scale for the objective rating of verbal and physical aggression. Am J Psychiatry 143:35–39, 1986

Zemlan FP, Hirschowitz J, Sautter FJ, et al: Impact of lithium therapy on core psychotic symptoms of schizophrenia. Br J Psychiatry 144:64–69, 1984

CHAPTER 9

Substance Abuse in Patients With Schizophrenia

Douglas Ziedonis, M.D., M.P.H.
Connie Nickou, Psy.D.

Substance abuse is the most common comorbidity among individuals with schizophrenia, and it worsens the prognosis and course of treatment. Substance use is to schizophrenia as lighter fluid is to fire. Consequently, comorbid substance abuse has a substantial impact on the lives of individuals with schizophrenia. The relationship between schizophrenia and substance abuse is complex. One component of the complexity is the heterogeneity of this dual-diagnosis subtype, determined in part by the specific substance(s) abused, the severity of the disorders, and the patient's motivation to deal with either problem.

Each type of substance has a unique pharmacological effect that can modify cognition, thought, and mood. Most substances interact with psychiatric medications that are used to treat schizophrenia through pharmacokinetic and/or pharmacodynamic interactions. In this chapter, we review the impact of specific substances of abuse as it relates to schizophrenia and examine the factors that relate to the onset and maintenance of substance abuse in this population and the implications for treatment.

In individuals with schizophrenia, substance use quickly progresses to abuse or dependence. The addictive disorder is a behavioral disorder with biopsychosocial-spiritual consequences, including medical, legal, vocational, social, family, and psychological problems. Even with abstinence, there is an underlying substance use disorder to address.

The underlying neurobiology of addictions is associated with the mesolimbic dopamine pathway. Reinforcement, pleasure, and reward are thought to be related to this pathway, with a focus on the ventral tegmentum area and nucleus accumbens. In this model, dopamine release results in pleasure and reward. Multiple pathways, including endogenous opioids, influence this process.

Motivation to enter substance abuse treatment and to stop using substances are important prognostic and treatment-matching factors in this population. Unfortunately, most dually diagnosed patients with schizophrenia have low motivation to stop using substances, and these patients require new and innovative interventions. Treatment strategies to manage the low- and higher-motivated dually diagnosed patients are described in this chapter. These include encouraging clinicians to develop realistic treatment goals and using treatment-matching strategies that take into account the motivational level to quit substance use.

Treating negative symptoms may be a critical factor in managing dually diagnosed patients. Negative symptoms appear to be affected by substance use and withdrawal. Individuals with schizophrenia may be self-medicating negative symptoms, including poor attention, anhedonia, and asociality. Providing effective treatment of both positive and negative symptoms of schizophrenia is of primary importance in treating the dually diagnosed patient.

Patients with a dual diagnosis of schizophrenia and substance abuse can be difficult to engage in treatment and are often revolving-door clients. They have numerous brief psychotic relapses that result in frequent emergency room visits and psychiatric hospitalizations. The dually diagnosed patient responds poorly to traditional psychiatric or substance treatment. Treating the schizophrenia patient with a comorbid substance use disorder calls for a new clinical perspective and requires mental health clinicians to learn new clinical approaches.

In addition, traditional substance abuse treatment approaches must be modified and integrated within traditional mental health treatment, including Motivational Enhancement Therapy (MET), relapse prevention therapy, community reinforcement approaches, 12-Step recovery, and pharmacotherapies for detoxification, protracted abstinence, and maintenance. In this chapter, we review the Motivation Based Dual Diagnosis Treatment (MBDDT) model, which offers a method for integrating the substance abuse treatment techniques into mental health treatment. The first step is to detect and diagnose the comorbid substance use disorder.

Definition of and Diagnostic Criteria for Substance Abuse

Detecting substance use and establishing a diagnosis among individuals with schizophrenia are carried out by asking clients about their use of substances, talking with collaterals (e.g., family, friends, other staff), obtaining urine toxicology screenings, and using substance abuse screening tools such as the CAGE questionnaire (Mayfield et al. 1974). Unfortunately, many clinicians fail to detect or recognize substance abuse in patients diagnosed with schizophrenia (Shaner et al. 1993). One reason is that psychiatric patients tend to have more severe consequences from smaller amounts of substance use than nonpsychiatric patients, and clinicians may be lulled into a false sense of security by focusing solely on the amount of substance use reported. A diagnosis of substance abuse is defined not by the amount or frequency of use, but rather by the consequences of use.

The diagnostic criteria of substance use disorders are outlined in DSM-IV (American Psychiatric Association 1994). Among psychiatric patients, one of the most salient clues to whether a patient has a substance abuse problem is continued use of the substance despite adverse consequences such as persistent or recurrent legal, financial, physical, psychological, or family problems. However, patients often minimize their substance-related problems and attribute those problems to other causes. The common consequences of illegal activity, episodic homelessness, poor treatment compliance, episodes of violent behavior, and multiple recurrent hospitalizations are important clues to substance abuse even when use is denied or minimized.

The impact of undiagnosed substance abuse in psychotic patients appears to worsen the course of their illness (Ananth et al. 1989). Clearly, the problem of undiagnosed substance abuse is more likely to change the course of treatment than diagnostic uncertainty within mental health settings; however, a discussion about dealing with diagnostic uncertainty is warranted.

Diagnostic Uncertainty in the Presence of Psychotic Symptoms and Substance Use

Even among the most experienced clinicians, establishing whether an individual has schizophrenia or a substance-induced psychotic disorder can be difficult because substances alone can induce or maintain the psychotic symptoms. For example, the effects of cocaine can mimic the psychotic symptoms of schizophrenia or other psychiatric symptoms such as depression, anxiety, and mania. Moreover, substance-using patients can be poorly compliant with taking their medication, and the presenting psychotic relapse may be due to noncompliance. The patient's specific clinical presentation is dependent on many factors, including the particular substance being used, the dose, the duration of use, the individual's tolerance for the substance, the period of time since the last dose, the expectations of the individual as to the substance's effects, and the environment or setting in which the substance is taken. The clinical presentation varies according to the different states of substance use: intoxication, withdrawal, or chronic usage (Ziedonis 1992).

Shaner et al. (1993) reported substantial diagnostic uncertainty in a longitudinal diagnosis study of 165 patients with chronic psychosis and cocaine abuse. This clinical research group attempted to establish the primary diagnosis by determining whether the client met DSM-III-R criteria for a psychotic disorder and not just isolated substance-induced psychotic symptoms. Information was gathered from all available sources, and ongoing assessments were conducted with a hope of having 6 weeks of abstinence to conclusively diagnose a non-substance-induced psychotic disorder. Shaner et al. found that a definitive diagnosis could not be established in most cases (93%) because of insufficient abstinence (78%), poor memory (24%), and/or inconsistent reporting by the patient (20%). To address the problems of poor memory and inconsistent reporting, Shaner et al. (1993) gathered additional information from clinical charts and significant others (e.g., family, friends, other staff).

Other helpful information from these sources includes assessing the age at onset of substance abuse relative to the onset of psychotic symptoms, assessing the temporal relationship of substance use and psychotic symptoms, and assessing family history. In the case of diagnostic uncertainty, a substance-induced disorder might be suggested when the client has a substantial family history for substance abuse, an early age at onset of substance abuse (particularly cocaine or amphetamine abuse), or the presence of psychotic symptoms mostly after substance use.

The problem of continued substance use during the assessment period was the most common reason for diagnostic uncertainty in the Shaner et al. (1993) study. According to DSM criteria, the diagnosis of schizophrenia should not be given if the presenting symptoms are due to the direct physiological effects of a substance (American Psychiatric Association 1994). However, the presentation of cocaine intoxication may be similar to the psychotic symptoms of schizophrenia. Signs and symptoms of intoxication sometimes may persist for hours or days beyond when the substance is detectable in body fluids. Although most substances and their metabolites clear the urine within 48 hours of ingestion, certain metabolites may be present for a longer period in chronic users. Satel and Lieberman (1991) maintain that a cocaine psychosis that persists for more than several days is indicative of an underlying psychotic disorder.

Persistent or increasing psychosis after 1 week of abstinence from cocaine suggests the need to treat the psychosis with medications. Shaner et al. (1993) suggest instituting concurrent treatment of both disorders in the context of diagnostic uncertainty.

The Shaner et al. study highlights the need to make clinical decisions even in the context of diagnostic uncertainty. After several months of abstinence, the risks and benefits of discontinuing the antipsychotic on a trial basis to further evaluate the diagnostic uncertainty issue might be considered with some individuals.

We now review the clinical epidemiology of substance abuse among individuals with schizophrenia as it relates to program development and clinical treatment needs.

Clinical Epidemiology of Comorbid Substance Use and Abuse

Although there is some variability because of sampling differences and use of different assessment instruments, the reported rates of comorbid substance abuse by individuals with schizophrenia have been uniformly high. As in the general population, the five substances most commonly used by individuals with schizophrenia are caffeine, nicotine, alcohol, marijuana, and cocaine. The Epidemiologic Catchment Area (ECA) study, with a population-based sample, reported lifetime rates of substance use disorders among individuals with schizophrenia of 47%, including about 34% for alcohol use disorders and approximately 28% for other drug use disorders (Regier et al. 1990). In mental health treatment settings, the current substance abuse rates range from 40% to 80%, and polysubstance abuse is common (Dixon et al. 1990; Schneier and Siris 1987; Ziedonis and Fisher 1996). A study at the Connecticut Mental Health Center found that 45% of outpatients with schizophrenia or a schizoaffective disorder had a current substance use disorder, including 35% who were abusing alcohol, 20% who were abusing cocaine, and 15% who were abusing marijuana. Most (77%) of these dually diagnosed patients had low motivation to stop using substances, and the level of motivation varied according to the specific substance of abuse (Ziedonis and Trudeau 1997).

Substance abuse is associated with being male, young, single or divorced, poorly educated, and depressed. Ironically, dually diagnosed patients with schizophrenia often have a higher level of premorbid social functioning before the onset of schizophrenia than non–dually diagnosed patients with schizophrenia.

Compared with individuals with schizophrenia who do not have a substance use disorder, individuals with schizophrenia and a substance use disorder have an earlier onset of alcohol/drug use and schizophrenia (Ziedonis 1992). A substance use disorder is more common when substance use begins prior to the onset of schizophrenia (Mueser and Gingerich 1994). Alcohol and nicotine are typically the first substances to be experimented with and used regularly and are considered to be gateway substances to marijuana, cocaine, and other illicit drugs.

Delaying the onset of use of these substances appears to reduce the likelihood that individuals will develop substance use disorders and experiment with illicit substances. Numerous patients admit to hallucinogen and marijuana abuse in their late adolescence and near the onset of their psychotic disorder. Some patients will attribute their mental illness to this exposure. Recently, MDMA (methylenedioxymethamphetamine; ecstacy) has become popular among adolescents and young adults. MDMA is known to destroy serotonin cells. Research has not clearly linked the cause of schizophrenia to illicit drug experimentation.

Impact of Substance Use on the Course of Schizophrenia

The impact of substance abuse on individuals with schizophrenia results from the combination of the pharmacological effects of the substances, the interactions (both pharmacokinetic and pharmacodynamic) of the substances and schizophrenia medication, and the behavioral consequences of the substance use disorder. This combination has biological, psychological, social, and spiritual consequences. Compared with non–dually diagnosed patients, dually diagnosed patients have a poorer prognosis, which includes increased hospitalizations, increased resource consumption, increased medication dosages, poorer medication compliance, increased vulnerability to social dysfunction, and increased suicide attempts. Substance use invariably exacerbates psychiatric symptoms. Persons with a dual diagnosis have more presentations at hospital emergency rooms; they also have more psychosocial problems, including housing problems and homelessness, poor nutrition, and financial problems (Westermeyer 1992).

Just as neuroleptics changed the clinical course of schizophrenia, one might predict that the chronic use of illicit drugs will also change the course and psychiatric symptoms of schizophrenia for the dually diagnosed patient. Careful and detailed descriptions of patterns of substance abuse and associated clinical effects may suggest further meaningful sub-types of dually diagnosed individuals with schizophrenia.

Initially, substances usually exacerbate and worsen psychiatric symptoms; however, some psychiatric symptoms may be reduced. The effect that substances have on psychiatric symptoms depends on the type of substance, the route of administration, the setting of drug usage, and the state of drug use (intoxication/withdrawal).

Positive and Negative Symptoms

Substance use appears to alter positive and negative symptoms acutely. The effect of chronic substance usage is less certain. Some studies found lower levels of negative symptoms (Dixon et al. 1990; Serper et al. 1995; Ziedonis et al. 1994); however, other studies found no difference in negative or positive symptoms (Zisook et al. 1992). Although stimulants can acutely improve mood and reduce anxiety in some patients (Brady et al. 1990), most individuals experience increased psychotic symptoms, mood lability, and insomnia (Dixon et al. 1990, Negrete et al. 1986).

Neuropsychological Functioning

Several studies have reported that substance abuse adversely affects neurocognitive functioning among individuals with schizophrenia, resulting in reduced attention and memory (Oepen et al. 1993; Sevy et al. 1990; Tracy et al. 1995). More research is needed to assess whether the effects of substance abuse on neuropsychological functioning are a temporary consequence of substance use or a more permanent, long-lasting result. In one study conducted among a nonpsychiatric sample, the investigators reported a significant correlation between stimulant abuse and a pattern of neurocognitive impairment, noting specific deficits noted in the areas of concentration, memory, nonverbal problem solving, and abstracting ability (O'Malley et al. 1992). Reducing substance use may improve cognitive functioning status.

Medication Effectiveness, Blood Levels, and Side Effects

Substances have a direct pharmacological effect on the central nervous system (CNS) that results in certain changes in cognition, thought, and mood. In addition, the effectiveness of medications can change because of pharmacodynamic and pharmacokinetic interactions. Substances can modify medication blood levels and the severity of side effects. Also, medication compliance is poor among dually diagnosed patients with low motivation to stop using substances. The metabolism of medications can be altered by hepatic damage caused by substances (alcohol, toxins, and intravenous drugs) and to direct competition/induction of the cytochrome P450 system. Both tobacco and caffeine increase the metabolism of certain medications.

All patients receiving neuroleptic medication are vulnerable to developing certain side effects. For example, tardive dyskinesia is an iatrogenic disorder affecting 20%–30% of psychiatric patients exposed to neuroleptics, and there is no effective treatment (Glazer and Morgenstern 1988). Research suggests that substance abuse is associated with earlier and more severe cases of tardive dyskinesia (Brady et al. 1990). In one study, patients who abused alcohol alone (25.4%) or alcohol in combination with cannabis (26.7%) were diagnosed with significantly higher rates of tardive dyskinesia compared with patients who abused sedatives, opioids, or stimulants (Olivera et al. 1990). Some substances/toxins can increase anticholinergic side effects and sedation side effects of medications.

Medical complications resulting from substance abuse and the various routes of administration can further impact psychiatric symptoms, medication dosages, and medication side effects.

Medical Problems

Substance abuse can result in poor physical and mental hygiene (often including poor eating, nutrition, and sleeping habits), liver disease (due to the metabolism of toxic substances), cardiac disease, risk of abscesses (infections from reactions to toxic substances being used to cut the drug), and reduced blood flow to the frontal cortex (often resulting in specific or diffuse neurological deficits). Other related medical problems involve the risk of exposure to HIV, either through sharing needles during intravenous drug abuse or through unprotected sexual activity. Some patients prostitute to support their drug habits, thereby increasing their risk of contracting sexually transmitted diseases.

Specific Substances and Their Impact

Specific substances vary in their neurobiological effects, symptoms, and addictive potential. The route of administration of the substance is another important factor. In this section, we review the impact of specific substances of abuse.

Caffeine

Caffeine intake is very prevalent among patients with schizophrenia; however, research on the effects of caffeine use is limited. Approximately 80%–

90% of individuals with schizophrenia consume caffeine daily (Test et al. 1989). Caffeine intake is associated with greater use of other substances and medications, especially cigarettes, benzodiazepines, and sedative-hypnotics (Greden et al. 1981).

Coffee and tea alter the absorption and metabolism of psychiatric medication because caffeine is metabolized in the liver by the cytochrome P450 system. Of note, smoking increases the metabolism of caffeine. Caffeine is an adenosine antagonist that increases second messengers for norepinephrine (Stahl 1996).

Caffeine use can increase alertness, vigilance, and ability to perform complex motor functions and can decrease fatigue. However, intoxication can lead to nervousness, restlessness, insomnia, tachycardia, palpitations, dry mouth, agitation, mild paranoia, and, after prolonged use, more severe symptoms of toxicity. Individuals develop tolerance to caffeine and develop withdrawal symptoms with abstinence. Although some patients report improvements in alertness and concentration, Hamera et al. (1995) found a strong relationship between reports of distress and caffeine use.

Nicotine

Nicotine dependence is very common among persons with schizophrenia—at least 50% and as much as 90% of individuals with schizophrenia smoke tobacco. This rate is much higher than the rate in the general population (27%) and significantly higher than rates for some other psychiatric disorders. Current smokers tend to be younger and more often male and have a larger number of psychiatric hospitalizations, higher rates of other substance abuse, and an earlier onset of schizophrenia than nonsmokers (Glassman 1993; Ziedonis et al. 1994).

Nicotine affects both the cholinergic system and the dopaminergic system (Hall 1980). Nicotine's primary effect on the cholinergic system can modulate dopamine activity. Nicotine's pharmacological effect can modify psychiatric symptoms and enhance attention and memory. Cigarette smoking alters the pharmacokinetics of antipsychotic medication metabolism.

Cigarette smoking is an important cytochrome P450 1AC inducer and increases drug clearance of many psychiatric medications by inducing hepatic microsomal enzymes. The "tar" (polynuclear aromatic hydrocarbons) in cigarettes, not the nicotine, causes this effect (Ziedonis and George 1997). The increase in metabolism requires that physicians prescribe significantly higher levels of neuroleptic medication for smokers than for nonsmokers, and smoking is known to decrease the blood levels of haloperidol, fluphenazine, thiothixene, clozapine, and olanzapine (Ereshefsky 1996; Ereshefsky et al. 1991). Abstinence from smoking increases neuroleptic, benzodiazepine, and antidepressant medication blood levels.

Several studies have assessed the impact of smoking on psychopathology. Ziedonis et al. (1994) compared 269 outpatients with schizophrenia or schizoaffective disorder according to their smoking status. Current smokers had significantly higher levels of positive symptoms than nonsmokers, and heavy smokers had the highest rate of positive symptoms. Heavy smokers had significantly fewer negative symptoms than nonsmokers/ light smokers. Goff et al. (1992) found, among patients with schizophrenia, that smokers had higher levels of both positive and negative symptoms compared with nonsmokers and no differences in levels of depression. Hamera et al. (1995) found that individuals with schizophrenia who decreased their nicotine use reported significantly higher levels of prodromal psychotic symptoms. Longitudinal studies are needed to better understand the complex relationship of nicotine use and psychopathology.

Sandyk (1993) investigated the relationship of smoking to the severity of cognitive impairment and found that among 111 persons with schizophrenia, smokers had significantly less cognitive impairment than nonsmokers. The author suggested that the high prevalence of smoking among schizophrenia patients may relate to the enhancing effects of nicotine on arousal, attention, and memory functions. Medications that are more effective in reducing negative symptoms may help improve these cognitive deficits and ameliorate the self-medication need to continue cigarette smoking.

Several studies have found that patients with schizophrenia who were switched from traditional neuroleptics to clozapine had a substantial reduction in their cigarette smoking without any specific nicotine dependence treatment or patient interest in stopping smoking (George et al. 1995; McEvoy et al. 1995). Although the mechanism underlying this reduction in nicotine use is unknown, neurobiological relationships between clozapine, negative symptoms, and nicotine receptors on dopamine tracts that connect to the frontal lobe suggest a plausible mechanism underlying the use of nicotine as self-medication of negative symptoms. Better treatment of negative symptoms may account for decreased need to self-medicate with nicotine. An equally plausible mechanism underlying these findings is the result of pharmacokinetic/pharmacodynamic interactions between nicotine and clozapine.

Alcohol

Alcohol use disorders are common among individuals with schizophrenia, occurring in 25%–50% of this population. Alcohol abuse and dependence are associated with unemployment, rural residence, lower educational level, and lower socioeconomic status in this population, although it is often difficult to separate cause from effect (Cuffel 1992).

Although older individuals tend to consume only alcohol and to use it in isolation (Cohen and Henkin 1995), polysubstance abuse is common among those who abuse alcohol (Drake and Wallach 1989; Ziedonis and Trudeau 1997). The likelihood of having severe alcohol dependence and polysubstance abuse increases with a family history of alcohol abuse (Noordsy et al. 1994). Some individuals use alcohol to alleviate the unwanted effects of other substances (e.g., cocaine, amphetamines, marijuana). The often combined use of alcohol and cocaine results in the development of a new cocaine metabolite that has been labeled coc-ethylene (McCance et al. 1995). This metabolite appears to lengthen the cocaine high and to increase the acute risks for cardiac disorders.

Alcohol is a depressant that usually initially has a calming effect but subsequently can lead to impaired thoughts and judgment. Alcohol intoxication and withdrawal can cause and exacerbate severe psychiatric symptoms and can be life threatening. The interaction between alcohol and medications can be lethal. Patients should be encouraged to avoid alcohol when using many of the psychiatric medications, including sedatives, hypnotics, sedating neuroleptics, and medications to treat pain, flu symptoms, allergies, and motion sickness. The symptoms resulting from combining alcohol and these medications can range from increased sedation to orthostatic hypotension to motor and intellectual impairment to coma to death. Psychotic symptoms are common in severe alcohol withdrawal, delirium tremens, alcohol amnestic disorder (Korsakoff's syndrome), alcoholic encephalopathy (Wernicke's syndrome), and alcohol hallucinosis.

Individuals with alcohol abuse and schizophrenia self-report using alcohol to reduce symptoms of anxiety, insomnia, and depression. However, these individuals are also more likely to manifest hostile threats, antisocial behaviors, paranoia, incoherent speech, depression, and suicidal thoughts than are non–alcohol abusers (Drake et al. 1989; Strakowski et al. 1994). Although some patients with chronic auditory hallucinations report that abusing alcohol is a temporary escape from the voices (Mueser and Gingerich 1994), alcohol use appears to exacerbate the positive and negative symptoms of schizophrenia (Brady et al. 1990). Frederick and Cotanch

(1995) found that, in particular, patients whose auditory hallucinations were of a hostile nature tended to use alcohol.

Chronic alcohol abuse can cause multiple medical consequences, including blackouts, gastritis, ulcers, cardiac disease, pancreatitis, hypoglycemia, muscle weakness, anemia, seizures, trauma, and liver disease. Heavy alcohol use interferes with the digestion and absorption of food, resulting in poor nutritional states. Alcohol's effect on the liver can also alter the metabolism of medications.

Marijuana

Marijuana use is common among individuals with schizophrenia (DeQuardo et al. 1994) and increases the risk for other drug abuse and psychiatric comorbidities. Marijuana is often the vehicle for abusing other illicit substances such as phencyclidine (PCP), amphetamines/cocaine, heroin, and formaldehyde (a neurotoxin).

Marijuana acts as a dopamine reuptake blocker and increases dopamine synthesis by increasing tyrosine hydroxylase activity (Gardner et al. 1990). Like antiparkinsonism drugs, marijuana also acts as an anticholinergic agent and consequently may be used in an attempt to relieve extrapyramidal side effects of medication. Unfortunately, marijuana use may actually increase the risk for tardive dyskinesia (Zaretsky et al. 1993). Marijuana may also reduce the effectiveness of neuroleptic medication (Knudsen and Vilmar 1984).

Although some patients may enjoy the marijuana high, marijuana use is associated with adverse psychological effects, including impaired short-term memory, amotivational syndrome, and depression. Marijuana use may also increase symptoms of anxiety and paranoia. Negrete et al. (1986) observed that persons with schizophrenia who used marijuana reported increased frequency of delusions and hallucinations.

Cocaine

Current rates of cocaine abuse or dependence are estimated to be between 15% and 37% among persons with schizophrenia. The use of cocaine dramatically increased with the easy access to "crack" cocaine. Crack cocaine comes prepackaged and ready to use and is widely available, relatively inexpensive, and extremely addictive. Individuals cook and then inhale crack to obtain an immediate "high," and this produces extremely elevated blood levels of cocaine. Cocaine hydrochloric acid is snorted by the addicted individual, whereas freebase or crack cocaine is inhaled. The inhaled route (similar to the intravenous route) results in a faster drug absorption rate and a higher peak blood level than the intranasal route of administration.

Cocaine is a dopamine agonist, and chronic cocaine use may lead to a supersensitivity of dopamine receptors. Chronic cocaine use causes a dopamine depletion state.

Cocaine is a powerful stimulant and may produce feelings of euphoria, alertness, heightened sexuality, a sense of well-being, and increased energy. Cocaine use can lead to physiological problems, including severe hypertension, sexual impotence, seizures, CNS damage, respiratory collapse, cardiac arrest, and stroke. Cocaine use also appears to exacerbate the positive symptoms of schizophrenia (Janowsky and Davis 1976).

Cocaine-abusing persons with schizophrenia are often younger at time of first psychiatric hospitalization, and their illness is more likely to be of the paranoid type (Lysaker et al. 1994). They have significantly higher hospitalization rates and more suicidal ideation and require higher medication dosages than other substance-using or nonusing schizophrenia patients (Seibyl et al. 1993).

The cycle of cocaine use and withdrawal may exacerbate feelings of depression and anhedonia. After a cocaine run or binge, users commonly experience a rebound dysphoria called a "cocaine crash" (Ziedonis et al. 1992). During these periods, individuals typically experience intense feelings of fatigue, listlessness, insomnia, and depression and are also at higher risk of developing suicidal ideation. The magnitude and duration of anhedonia may be proportional to the amount of cocaine consumed (Markou and Koob 1991).

Etiological Factors in Substance Abuse

Biological, psychological, and social factors have a role in the development of a substance use disorder among individuals with schizophrenia. A better understanding of these factors may lead to improvements in prevention, early diagnosis, and treatment.

Biological Factors

From a biological perspective, the dopaminergic system appears to play an important role in both schizophrenia and substance use disorders. Brain regions suspected of influencing reinforcement and reward include the ventral tegmentum area and the nucleus accumbens. The ventral tegmental area is linked to the prefrontal cortex, which some research has hypothesized may be hypoactive in schizophrenia (Glassman 1993). Substances of abuse may be especially reinforcing in individuals with schizophrenia because of the combined stimulation of subcortical brain reward mechanisms and prefrontal cortex.

Evidence of a genetic risk factor was found in a twin study of individuals with comorbid alcohol abuse and schizophrenia (Kendler 1985). Obtaining a family history may help in early detection of substance abuse and in targeting substance abuse prevention strategies.

Substance abuse may either cause schizophrenia or precipitate schizophrenia in individuals who are genetically vulnerable. Andreasson et al. (1987) found higher rates of a history of marijuana use in persons who later developed schizophrenia. Ballenger and Post (1978) hypothesized that repeated alcohol abuse produces a kindling-like effect on the brain and that the individual becomes vulnerable to develop psychiatric symptoms from any amount of alcohol.

Psychological Factors

Psychological factors have an important role in the initiation and maintenance of substance use and abuse. Persons with schizophrenia self-report using substances for pleasure, to alleviate boredom, to connect socially, and to cope with persistent symptoms of their illness (Mueser et al. 1995).

The *self-medication theory* suggests that individuals with schizophrenia may use drugs to self-medicate depressive disorder, including postpsychotic depression, negative symptoms of schizophrenia, and neuroleptic side-effect symptoms (Khantzian 1985). Some patients report feeling less dysphoric, less anxious, and more energetic while intoxicated (Dixon et al. 1990). Schneier and Siris (1987) found that while groups of individuals with schizophrenia used significantly more amphetamines, cocaine, cannabis, hallucinogens, inhalants, caffeine, and nicotine compared with control groups, their use of alcohol, opiates, and sedative-hypnotics was significantly less than or the same as that of the control groups. Studies of patients' reasons for using drugs may help in delineating subtypes within the dually diagnosed population.

Social Factors

Social changes have increased the availability of and access to alcohol, nicotine, and low-cost illicit drugs for the dually diagnosed population. For many individuals with a severe mental illness, substance use is a social activity that links them with non–mentally ill substance-abusing acquaintances and drug dates with sexual partners. A substance-abusing peer group serves to normalize the substance abuse behavior and also exposes the mentally ill individual to new problems.

Deinstitutionalization, social programs, and entitlements for individuals with schizophrenia have increased the accessibility of substances. Community social programs and housing often exist with limited support and supervision. These changes, along with patients' desire for social contact and patients' participation in various social groups, have led to an increase in substance abuse for some patients with chronic mental illness (Westermeyer 1992).

Furthermore, substances produce relatively instantaneous effects for patients, whereas finding other sources of enjoyment requires more time. In fact, some psychiatric patients may actually prefer, for reasons of social acceptability, being labeled an alcoholic or drug addict to being labeled schizophrenic or mentally ill (Ziedonis 1995).

Although disability income is provided with the intent to help patients pay for basic needs, this source of funding may be diverted to purchase substances. Shaner et al. (1993) studied the temporal patterns of cocaine use, psychiatric symptoms, and psychiatric hospitalization in a sample of 105 male cocaine-abusing veterans with schizophrenia. The patients were receiving disability income weekly. The researchers found that cocaine use, psychiatric symptoms, and hospital admissions all peaked during the first week of the month—soon after the receipt of the disability check. The average patient in the study spent about one-half his income on illicit drugs. The consequences of this diversion of funds resulted in depletion of funds needed for housing and food, exacerbation of psychiatric symptoms, more frequent psychiatric hospitalizations, and a high rate of homelessness. The potential implications are clear. Strategies for helping patients manage their disability income need to be considered in the early phases of treatment planning.

Patient Assessment and Differential Diagnosis

An initial substance abuse assessment should be completed for every patient in mental health treatment settings (Table 9–1). However, even when all patients are asked, some patients will completely deny any usage, and only urine toxicology screening or information from significant others will detect use.

Patterns of Use

Questions about current and past patterns of substance use should cover, among other items, frequency and amount of use, route(s) of administration, periods of most intensive use, use changes during the month, last use

---

Table 9–1. Assessing substance use and abuse in patients with psychiatric disorders

---

1. Ask about patterns of usage (e.g., specific amounts, frequency, last use, route of administration).
2. Obtain a complete family history for both mental illness and substance abuse.
3. Screen for use and/or abuse (urine/breath toxicology and use of CAGE questionnaires and other tools).
4. Assess for common consequences of substance abuse (especially legal problems, episodes of homelessness, recurrent brief hospitalizations, and poor treatment compliance).
5. Ask about the patient's perception of the benefits for continued use and his or her reasons to quit using the substance, and establish the patient's current motivational level to quit using each substance.
6. Assess previous substance abuse or dual-diagnosis treatment episodes, inquiring about what the treatment included and how well the patient responded.

---

of each substance, and the combination and temporal sequence of substances used. Substances to be screened for include alcohol, nicotine, caffeine, prescription medications, inhalants, formaldehyde, and other illicit drugs (Ziedonis and Fisher 1994). The use of a time line can help organize the assessment. With important life events used as anchor points, the time line should include the age at onset of use for each substance and the progression from use to problem use to dependence. The psychiatric history can be transposed onto the time line to help the clinician to begin to understand potential relationships between the substance abuse and psychiatric symptoms.

Asking about last substance use is helpful in determining which type of withdrawal symptoms to expect and in assessing the need for detoxification. The patient's psychiatric presentation may vary according to the type(s) of substance and the substance use states of intoxication, withdrawal, or chronic use. For example, the effects of cocaine withdrawal may appear similar to clinical depression in terms of dysphoric mood, suicidal ideation, nightmares, and psychomotor changes (Dilsaver 1987).

Urine/Breath Toxicology Screening

Urine toxicology and alcohol Breathalyzer tests are invaluable tools in the assessment of all patients and in the monitoring of response to dual-diagnosis treatment. Denial of substance use is common. One study found that one-third of the individuals with schizophrenia who came to the emergency room were recent cocaine users; of this group, 50% reported that they had not used cocaine recently (Shaner et al. 1993).

Urine testing is helpful in estimating the time of last use of a substance. Cocaine (or its metabolite benzoylecgonine) is usually present in the urine for only 2–3 days; however, tests for cocaine among heavy users can remain positive for up to 1 week of abstinence. In contrast, marijuana is fat soluble and may be detected for as long as 4–6 weeks in the daily user.

Screening for Substance Abuse

The use of substance abuse screening instruments can increase the clinician's suspiciousness of a substance use disorder. Examples of such instruments include the CAGE questionnaire and the Michigan Alcoholism Screening Test (MAST; Seltzer 1971). Although these instruments can be helpful in the clinical population of dually diagnosed schizophrenia patients (Kofoed 1991), more research is needed to evaluate these instruments and to develop alternative instruments for this population.

Another screening clue for substance abuse is the number of cigarettes smoked by the patient. Compared with nonsmokers, heavy smokers (those smoking >25 cigarettes per day) are three to four times more likely to have other substance use disorders (Glassman 1993; Ziedonis et al. 1994).

Common Consequences of Substance Abuse

The presence of common consequences of substance abuse increases the likelihood of an existing substance use disorder. Such consequences include episodes of homelessness, legal problems, verbal threats, violence, noncompliance with treatment, need for higher dosages of neuroleptics, multiple medical problems, frequent emergency room visits, multiple psychiatric rehospitalizations in 1 year, suicidal ideation/suicide attempts, and crisis-prone lifestyles (Ziedonis and Fisher 1996).

History of Past Substance Abuse and Treatment

An initial evaluation should assess the history of past substance abuse and/or treatment, including what types of treatments were attempted and for how long. This is important for developing appropriate and realistic treatment planning.

Motivational Assessment

Persons with psychiatric disorders often have low motivation to quit using substances, and motivation to quit using varies according to substance (Ziedonis and Trudeau 1997). For example, the person may wish to stop using cocaine but not alcohol. However, since motivation to quit is a state, not a trait, reassessment must occur regularly. Patients may be willing to attend dual-diagnosis treatment but may not be committed to stop using substances.

Prochaska et al. (1992) described a motivational scale commonly used in the addiction treatment community. The scale consists of five stages: precontemplation, contemplation, preparation, action, and maintenance. In the *precontemplation* stage, the patient continues to use substances and denies or minimizes the use and associated problems. In the *contemplation* stage, the patient continues to use the substance but now admits that continued use is problematic and he or she is ambivalent about stopping the substance use in the distant future. Patients in the precontemplation or contemplation stages have low motivation and are unlikely to change their behavior soon without a strong external lever. In the *preparation* stage, the patient continues to use the substance but is now interested in stopping use during the next month and needs help to develop a plan to achieve this goal. In the *action* stage, the patient is willing to and does participate in treatment in order to stop using the substance. In the *maintenance* stage, the patient has remained abstinent for 3–6 months.

Another method of assessing motivation requires the clinician to observe the patient's responsiveness to discussing his or her substance use. Typically, the more motivated patients are spontaneous and open about the negative consequences of their substance use. They may discuss previous substance abuse treatment and explain why they are more motivated now. Assessing the person's current level of motivation can facilitate the discovery of potential sources of external motivation, such as anticipated loss of housing, financial support, employment, family, marriage, and freedom from jail. External levers can be helpful in eliciting and maintaining change, including increasing internal motivation and achieving abstinence.

Dual Diagnosis Treatment Approaches

Treatment of dually diagnosed patients with schizophrenia requires addressing both the schizophrenia and the substance use disorders in a comprehensive, coordinated, and integrated manner. Psychosocial and medication treatments for both disorders must be integrated into the treatment plan. Treatment is linked in a system of care with housing, entitlements, rehabilitation, and community services. The specific type(s) of substance abused determines the adjunctive medications to be used for detoxification or managing the protracted abstinence phase.

In the past, treatment of comorbid substance abuse was not provided in the mental health treatment system, and the dually diagnosed patient was referred to addiction treatment programs for substance abuse treatment. Substance abuse treatment was sequential and nonintegrated for the higher-motivated clients and nonexistent for patients with low motivation. Mental health and addiction treatment systems engaged in turf battles, and as a result clinical outcomes were poor.

Recent Treatment Models

New models have been developed within the mental health system to integrate substance abuse treatment for the dually diagnosed, including the Assertive Community Treatment Team model (Drake et al. 1993), the Integrated Treatment model (Minkoff 1989), the Stages of Treatment model (Osher and Kofoed 1989), and the Motivation Based Dual Diagnosis Treatment model (Ziedonis and Fisher 1996). These models share similar clinical values, including an empathic approach, coordination of services, comprehensive services, case management, and outreach efforts. Integration of mental health and addiction treatment approaches is suggested to match the patient's stage of recovery and motivational level.

Assertive Community Treatment Team

The Assertive Community Treatment Team model (Drake et al. 1993) is a stage-wise, cognitive-behavioral substance abuse treatment integrated into comprehensive community mental health services that include outreach, case management, and medications. Multidisciplinary teams serve as the "primary clinician" for a relatively small number of patients and are involved in the patient's treatment in all settings. The teams are outpatient-oriented, and intensive case management is executed within the patient's natural environment. The model incorporates Osher and Kofoed's (1989) five stages of dual-diagnosis treatment: engagement, persuasion, coercion, relapse prevention, and action (which are similar to but different from the five motivational levels of Prochaska and DiClemente).

Integrated Treatment

The Integrated Treatment model (Minkoff 1989) emphasizes case-management care in an integrated manner that is based on the premise that there are parallels between the disorders of schizophrenia and substance abuse. Both disorders are chronic, relapsing conditions with biological underpinnings. Both illnesses are stigmatizing. Individuals often deny or minimize the presence or impact of both disorders. In this model, after a relapse to either condition occurs, a period of stabilization ensues prior to rehabilitation. An integrated model addresses both disorders simultaneously and recognizes the parallels between the two disorders.

Motivation Based Dual Diagnosis Treatment

The MBDDT model builds on the values and philosophy of the Integrated Treatment and Assertive Community Treatment Team models and matches clinical treatment approaches according to the type of psychiatric/substance use disorder, the severity of the disorder, and the patient's motivational level to address the addiction problem. MBDDT focuses on the addiction problem; more specifically, it offers a method for integrating substance abuse treatment techniques into mental health treatment. The model helps organize mental health staff training and treatment planning by suggesting specific substance abuse and dual-diagnosis treatment approaches.

In the MBDDT model, the patient's motivational level is determined on the basis of the five motivational stages of Prochaska et al. (1992) discussed earlier. Each stage is matched with specific treatment approaches from MET, 12-Step recovery approaches, medication strategies (for both the psychiatric and substance abuse problems), psychoeducation, social skills training, vocational rehabilitation, behavioral contracting, peer-support counseling, and family involvement. Additional treatment strategies include vocational exploration, self-care skills, sleep hygiene, case management, money management, and practical problem solving. Other social skills training might include continued focus on medication management, relationship skills, communication skills with medical personnel, transportation skills, grieving losses, expressing feelings, refusal/avoidance skills, stress management skills, and leisure skills (Nikkel 1994).

The three primary substance abuse treatment approaches that have been integrated into MBDDT are MET, relapse prevention (cognitive-behavioral therapy), and 12-Step recovery approaches. These three therapies are described in detail in the Project MATCH manuals that are available free of charge from the National Clearinghouse for Alcohol and Drug Information (1-800-729-6686; www.health.org).

In MBDDT, the patients with lower motivation receive more individual treatment, and their substance abuse treatment is integrated into mental health treatment groups. These groups increase patients' motivation through MET, problem solving, and improving relationships. Higher-motivated clients receive dual-diagnosis relapse prevention therapy (blending social skills training and addiction relapse prevention cognitive therapies), 12-Step recovery, and substance abuse medication treatments.

In the remainder of this chapter, we focus on the specific treatment approaches for both lower- and higher-motivated patients with schizophrenia.

Treatment for Lower-Motivated Patients

Clinicians commonly have unrealistic treatment goals and time expectations for patients with lower motivation to stop using substances. For example, individuals who minimize the impact of their substance use and who are not interested in quitting that use will be unlikely to achieve immediate abstinence. A more realistic and appropriate goal for clinicians is to help the person to recognize and acknowledge that there is a substance abuse problem and to establish a long-term commitment to engage in dual-diagnosis treatment.

In working with lower-motivated patients, the emphasis should be on the integration of substance abuse treatment into existing therapy groups. Poorly motivated patients are not interested in attending groups labeled "dual diagnosis." As a way to increase motivation, "healthy living groups" can be incorporated into treatment. These groups use MET and focus on practical discussions of healthy living, problem solving, and improving relationships. Treatment of the lower-motivated patient is an ongoing process and usually involves numerous relapses and slow movement—with the addition of multiple supports, external motivators, and monitors as needed—toward abstinence (Ziedonis and Trudeau 1997; Kofoed and Keys 1988).

In addition to the three primary substance abuse psychosocial approaches (MET, relapse prevention, and 12-Step facilitation), the Community Reinforcement Approach (CRA) is being evaluated in treating chronic psychiatric patients. CRA offers a way to develop external motivation for a population with limited external motivators. Disability income provides a real-world mechanism for exploring the behavior therapy principles of contingencies, rewards, and consequences. CRA is based on the behavior therapy principles of contingencies and rewards and links urine testing results with a voucher program. The entitlement system of payee conservator provides a mechanism by which to use CRA techniques and to help secure stable housing. The CRA approach supports the inclusion of lifestyle counseling that focuses on recreational counseling, social skills/assertiveness training, and educational counseling (Hellerstein et al. 1987; Higgins et al. 1994; Miller and Rollnick 1991). Continued research with this methodology may be effective in attempts to engage patients in treatment and to help them maintain some stable early abstinence.

Motivational Enhancement Therapy is an empathic and short-term goal-oriented approach in which the patient is viewed as self-directed and responsible for and capable of changing specific behaviors. The clinician helps to mobilize the patient's own inner resources. MET attempts to build motivation for change and to strengthen commitment to change. The clinician matches specific clinical techniques with the patient's particular motivational level. MET has been used in shaping a variety of behaviors, including improving compliance with medication treatment, addressing eating disorder problems, and exercising and engaging in healthier living activities.

In MET, patient resistance is seen as a problem with the therapist's approach in discussing the issue. For example, often the most difficult part of MET for clinicians is to refrain from providing advice, judgment, agreement/disagreement, solutions, or interpretations. However, an empathic approach often encourages the person to elicit self-motivational statements to consider stopping substance use. Using the MET "decisional balance" of comparing the pros and cons of their continued substance use and of stopping their substance use, lower-motivated patients will be more likely to discuss their reasons for continued use and the perceived benefits of use. Some may share their fears of quitting or their sense of hopelessness. General discussions with patients about areas that they are struggling with or that are important to them may lead to their reevaluating their current substance use.

At the end of a therapy session, the clinician might summarize what was discussed, provide feedback on the information discussed, and consider psychoeducation on relevant topics. Information might include the medical effects of the abused substance or how substance use can affect one's psychiatric condition. More detailed descriptions of MET techniques can be found in the literature (Miller and Rollnick 1991; Miller et al. 1992; National Institute on Alcohol Abuse and Alcoholism 1992; Project MATCH Research Group 1998).

Without external levers, individuals initially seen in the precontemplation stage will likely require years to evolve through an ambivalence to change, attempts at harm reduction, a commitment to quit using, and, finally, continued abstinence. Individuals in the precontemplation stage often benefit from receiving information and feedback related to the substance abuse problem. Clinicians should attempt to engage the person in an open and nonjudgmental manner to discuss his or her substance use. Treatment plans should state the motivational level and outline the immediate treatment goals and the specific techniques to be employed. Although the ultimate goal is directed toward abstinence, initial goals should emphasize harm reduction and focus on strengthening the commitment to change. The process of strengthening the commitment to change is a long-term effort toward continued abstinence.

As their motivation increases, individuals enter the contemplation stage and become willing to consider that a problem exists and that change may be possible. Although the patient has admitted to a problem, he or she also continues to be stuck in ambivalence. To move from contemplation to preparation, the patient must be able to generate enough factors to tip the "decisional balance" scale toward not using substances. In addition to affirming that change is difficult for all of us, the clinician may have the client complete the "decisional balance" sheet during a therapy session or as homework. The clinician should continue to look for self-motivational statements made by the patient. Clinicians should also consider the use of follow-up techniques such as letters and phone calls to ensure that patients keep treatment appointments.

Persons in preparation have decided to take steps to change their behavior. In this stage, the goal is to help the individual find a change plan that is acceptable, accessible, appropriate, and effective. Determining the person's strength of commitment is important. If the individual is willing to develop the plan, sign the plan, and then follow through on specific achievable goals, a high level of commitment has been indicated. Willingness to problem-solve about barriers to achieving his or her goals is another indicator of commitment. Fear of failure or success must be acknowledged. Successful achievement of planned goals allows additional successes to follow.

Family involvement and family education can be a critical component of treatment if the family is still involved with the patient. There are already many support groups for family members of substance abusers (e.g., Alanon, Cocanon), and groups specifically for family members of dually diagnosed individuals are being developed.

Medications for the Patient With Lower Motivation: Preparing for Dual Diagnosis Treatment

Medication treatment for dually diagnosed persons has some special considerations; however, the fundamental concepts for medication treatment of schizophrenia remain the same. In treating patients with lower motivation to stop substance use, the primary pharmacotherapy goals are to reduce the negative and positive symptoms of schizophrenia and to improve treatment compliance. Antipsychotic medications can help manage the positive and/or negative symptoms of schizophrenia. Dosing of these medications should be titrated to balance the benefits and risks of the medication, including improving effectiveness and reducing side effects. Improving the patient's motivation to maintain the prescribed medication regimen is important, and compliance can be improved by reducing the positive and negative symptoms of schizophrenia, providing psychoeducation, and/or using depot medication.

Two important pharmacotherapy considerations are the use of intramuscular injections of depot neuroleptic medication (i.e., haloperidol or fluphenazine) and the use of atypical neuroleptics (e.g., clozapine or risperidone). Injectable depot medication is an underutilized intervention that can guarantee medication compliance when administered. The depot neuroleptics help reduce the positive symptoms of schizophrenia and may increase participation in nonpharmacological interventions, thus reducing rates of psychotic relapse and rehospitalization. Haloperidol decanoate appears to have several advantages over fluphenazine decanoate, including a lower risk of extrapyramidal side effects (thereby requiring the use of less antiparkinsonism medications) and only once-per-month dosing frequency (every 4 weeks vs. every 2 weeks), resulting in fewer injections per year and reduced staff time requirements.

The atypical antipsychotic medications (the FDA approved clozapine in 1990, risperidone in 1994, olanzapine in 1996, and quetiapine in 1997) differ from traditional neuroleptic medications in demonstrating improved effectiveness in treating the negative symptoms of schizophrenia and having fewer extrapyramidal side effects. The atypical antipsychotics have a different receptor-binding profile, with an affinity for the serotonin receptors that may be important in the neurobiology of cocaine and alcohol dependence.

The atypical antipsychotics may be important in the treatment of dually diagnosed patients with low motivation to stop using because they offer specific advantages over the traditional neuroleptics, including improved efficacy in reducing negative symptoms and fewer side effects. Patients who may be attempting to self-medicate their negative symptoms or who experience an increase in symptoms during withdrawal may find the atypical antipsychotics especially helpful.

In animal studies, Kosten and Nestler (1994) compared haloperidol, clozapine, and vehicle during training and testing of cocaine place conditioning with rats. (In place conditioning, a rat is administered cocaine only in one chamber, even though the rat has equal access to two chambers. Usually the animal develops a strong preference to be in the chamber where the animal was able to access cocaine.) Administration of clozapine attenuated place conditioning to cocaine, whereas chronic administration of haloperidol enhanced place conditioning to cocaine. In other words, when receiving haloperidol, the rats preferred to stay in the area where they received cocaine, and the rats receiving clozapine avoided the cocaine area. Other studies, consistent with these findings, have found that clozapine partially attenuates the discriminating stimulus and self-administration effects of cocaine (Vanover et al. 1993).

Since clinical trials have not compared different atypical neuroleptics in the treatment of dually diagnosed individuals, selecting an atypical antipsychotic should be based on clinical experience and judgment. In this population, risperidone is a first-choice agent because it is not sedating and has low risk for extrapyramidal side effects at therapeutic dosages (4–6 mg). Olanzapine and clozapine have anticholinergic properties that increase the risk of dangerous symptoms when combined with alcohol. Preliminary studies and clinical experience support the efficacy of using the atypical antipsychotics for dually diagnosed schizophrenia patients and the need for further research in this area (Buckley et al. 1994).

Treatment for Higher-Motivated Patients

As patients move into the preparation phase and become more motivated, the focus begins to change. It is during this time that the clinician begins to shift the core therapy approach from MET to Dual Diagnosis Relapse Prevention (DDRP). DDRP is a time-limited, 6-month outpatient therapy approach designed specifically to help clients transition to the maintenance stage. DDRP is a hybrid cognitive-behavioral therapy that modifies and integrates substance abuse relapse prevention techniques and psychiatric social skills training. The focus is on developing general coping strategies and skills that may help prevent relapses and improve everyday functioning.

In DDRP, clinicians emphasize the need for effective communication and problem solving, the identification of early warning signs and high-risk situations, and the need to develop coping strategies and ways to structure one's day. The content of therapy sessions alternates emphasis between substance abuse and psychiatric problems and considers how each problem can affect the other one.

In developing an integrated approach, it is useful to monitor individual patients' progress and look for "windows of opportunity" to reinforce psychiatric or substance use issues. DDRP uses the behavior therapy approaches of *active role playing, modeling* (done by the clinician and/or another patient), *coaching* (when the clinician stands close and assists the client during a role play), the giving of *positive and negative feedback to their peers,* and the assignment of *homework.* Role-play techniques, including problem-solving skills and communication skills, can be introduced in group and/or individual therapy.

In DDRP, traditional relapse prevention therapy was modified to treat patients with schizophrenia who might have deficits in attention span, abstraction, reading, and social skills. Specific relapse-prevention techniques include assessing internal and external triggers, defining slips versus relapses, analyzing a relapse, developing coping and relaxation skills, carrying out drug refusal exercises, structuring time, managing a "slip," and understanding the abstinence violation effect (Ziedonis 1992). DDRP focuses on the problem of relapsing to substance use or psychosis and teaches skills that help individuals identify and cope with early warning signs or triggers.

In the past 5 years, DDRP has further evolved to integrate more 12-Step recovery language, spiritual awareness, and social support strategies. We now use the term *Dual Recovery Therapy* to describe the approach (Ziedonis et al. 2000).

The Process of Recovery

As patients progress in the recovery process, they develop extended periods of abstinence and are considered to be in the maintenance stage. The transition from action to maintenance can be difficult. During the maintenance stage, the focus shifts from just staying abstinent to improving core areas of one's life. For the nonschizophrenic substance abuser, this stage of addiction recovery has been labeled Stage II recovery (Larson 1985). The focus now should be on reducing self-defeating behaviors and decreasing involvement in dysfunctional relationships. Individuals begin attempting to pursue alternative "highs," including employment, healthier relationships with others, new recreational activities, exercise, and other social outlets with nonusers.

This transition phase can be more difficult for individuals with schizophrenia, and both clinicians and patients must remember that the learning process is ongoing, not finite. Relapse is always a possibility. Individuals may cycle through the motivational stages at various times in their lives. Old patterns may reemerge, and new stressors may bring on cravings and ineffective coping strategies. Stressors may include psychiatric symptoms as well as familial, legal, housing, and other problems. Sustaining change can be difficult, and positive patterns may need to be learned and relearned until the patient is able to fully integrate them into his or her life. Serving as peer counselors can facilitate this integration and help to reinforce the patient's motivation. Encouraging involvement in self-help groups at this time may be very appropriate, particularly 12-Step meetings that target dually diagnosed individuals such as those at mental health facilities.

Twelve-Step Programs

Although 12-Step recovery (e.g., Alcoholics Anonymous, Alanon) is usually an important aspect of treatment for most non–dually diagnosed substance abusers, clinical experience in referring individuals with schizophrenia to 12-Step programs has been mixed. The most effective use of 12-Step programs appears to occur when the meetings take place within a mental health setting or a community setting that is open and receptive to individuals with a mental illness. Many areas now have 12-Step meetings designed for persons with chronic mental illness, including Dual Recovery Anonymous and Double-Trudgers.

Clinicians must be aware of the stigmatization of medication and other misinformation that occurs at some 12-Step meetings and within some substance abuse treatment programs. Unfortunately, these factors have resulted in individuals receiving misguided advice to stop their psychiatric medications. Staff must also be aware of how they and the patient perceive the use of medication, and the message should be clear that medications are only one tool in the toolbox and are not magic bullets. The Alcoholics Anonymous publication *The AA Member: Medication and Other Drugs* provides support for the appropriate use of medications (Alcoholics Anonymous 1984; Ziedonis and Kosten 1991).

Medications for Higher-Motivated Patients: Targeting Specific Substances of Abuse

Medications that target specific substance use disorders are used for detoxification, craving reduction, and relief of protracted abstinence withdrawal symptoms and as agonist maintenance agents. Some of these medications may also help to reduce the negative symptoms of schizophrenia that in turn may improve the detoxification, protracted abstinence, and maintenance phases. Unfortunately, there have been limited pharmacotherapy trials for substance-abusing individuals with schizophrenia, despite increasing clinical experience in using these medications safely and effectively. Although traditional medications for substance abuse are clinically used in this population, randomized clinical trials have not been reported.

Alcohol Dependence

Adjunctive medications that are FDA approved for use in the treatment of alcohol use disorders include disulfiram (Antabuse) and naltrexone (ReVia). Disulfiram blocks the enzyme alcohol dehydrogenase and causes an acute reaction when alcohol is absorbed into the body—usually through drinking, though also through skin contact in extreme cases. Clinical experience is mixed in using this medication, and randomized controlled trials are lacking. Side effects of disulfiram include headache and sedation; however, the reaction between alcohol and disulfiram is the primary concern. Liver function tests should be assessed at baseline and continue to be monitored.

Naltrexone is an opiate receptor blocker most commonly used in treating opiate addiction. However, recent behavioral and pharmacological studies with both animals and humans suggest a link between the endogenous opiate system and alcohol misuse. Both naloxone and naltrexone decrease alcohol consumption in rats. In humans, naltrexone has been used as an effective pharmacological agent in the treatment of alcohol dependence (O'Malley et al. 1992) and has been shown to reduce alcohol consumption and lower rates of relapse when compared with placebo. Specifically, patients treated with naltrexone report fewer drinking days, fewer drinks consumed per occasion, and lower rates of relapse to heavy alcohol use. Clinical experience suggests that this medication can be used safely and may have some benefit in improving outcomes. The common side effects of naltrexone include nausea and sedation. As with disulfiram, liver function tests should be evaluated and monitored.

Early research had speculated that an opioid antagonist may help to reduce the psychotic symptoms of schizophrenia, but research to date has yielded mixed results. Naloxone did not improve symptoms in one sample of medicated schizophrenia patients (Naber et al. 1984), but another study found that naloxone significantly decreased levels of tension on the Brief Psychiatric Rating Scale (Lehman et al. 1979). These data suggest that naltrexone is well tolerated by individuals with schizophrenia and does not increase their psychiatric symptoms or interact with other psychiatric medications, including neuroleptics, lithium, and antidepressants (O'Malley et al. 1992).

Nicotine Dependence

Treatment guidelines for nicotine dependence have recently been developed (American Psychiatric Association 1996) and include multicomponent behavior therapy and adjunctive medications of transdermal nicotine patch, nicotine gum, nicotine spray, and clonidine. Several nicotine cessation studies for smokers with schizophrenia have been reported (George et al., in press; Ziedonis and George 1997). These studies found that intensive nicotine dependence treatment with both nicotine replacement and behavior therapy results in about 20% of patients maintaining abstinence for an extended period (6 months). Atypical antipsychotics may help improve nicotine dependence treatment for patients with schizophrenia. More clinical trials of cigarette smokers with schizophrenia are needed.

Cocaine Dependence

Few randomized clinical pharmacotherapy trials on cocaine dependence in patients with schizophrenia have been reported in the literature. Pharmacotherapy strategies in treating non–dually diagnosed cocaine abusers have focused on medications with specific dopaminergic activity that might reverse or compensate for the neurophysiological changes that result from chronic cocaine administration. Cocaine is a potent dopamine reuptake blocker with an acute effect of increasing activity in dopaminergic pathways, including endogenous reward systems. Chronic cocaine administration results in a supersensitization of presynaptic dopamine autoreceptors, which increases the threshold for activation of (and hence down-regulates) the dopaminergic system.

Numerous studies have evaluated the treatment of non–dually diagnosed cocaine abusers with dopamine reuptake blockers and dopamine agonists, and most of these studies did not find clinically significant improvements in outcomes. Of note, several studies suggest that the depressed cocaine abuser may benefit from antidepressants (Rao et al. 1995; Ziedonis et al. 1992). Recent studies of cocaine dependence in patients with schizophrenia have found adjunctive medications, including mazindol, desipramine, and imipramine, to provide limited additional benefit in reducing cocaine use (Ziedonis et al. 2000).

Substance Abuse Prevention Among Individuals With Schizophrenia

Given the high risk of developing a substance abuse comorbidity among individuals with schizophrenia, substance abuse prevention efforts might be aimed at primary prevention (to prevent the secondary disorder of substance abuse) and at secondary prevention (to do early detection and implementation of an intervention to stop the progression from use to abuse). The clinical epidemiology findings discussed in this chapter suggest opportunities for prevention programming. Part of the change can occur by changing the mental health system's attitude toward all addictions, including nicotine smoking.

Primary substance abuse prevention should target all individuals with schizophrenia, especially the younger patient and the patient who smokes cigarettes. Prevention efforts can be extended into the community support services of residential services, vocational programs, and social clubs. The use of prevention audiovisual materials, peer support programs, healthy coping skills development, and drug resistance skills training could all promote healthy relationships and nonchemical ways to improve one's well-being. Such programs could reinforce the cultural shift of addressing substance abuse problems and integrating treatment within a mental health setting (Ziedonis 1995).

Summary

Substance abuse is the most common comorbidity among individuals with schizophrenia and results in poor clinical outcomes and high use of costly services. Undetected substance abuse continues to be a major problem in mental health settings. After specialized training has been completed and realistic goals and expectations have been established, helping persons who are dually diagnosed can be challenging, rewarding, and effective.

Recovery is often a developmental process that requires time and incremental successes. Effective dual-diagnosis treatment provides integrative and comprehensive services, matches treatment to individual needs, and incorporates the strengths of all possible treatment philosophies, including motivational enhancement, traditional mental health approaches, 12-Step self-help recovery, the medical model, and appropriate use of pharmacological, behavioral, social, and prevention approaches.

The Motivation Based Dual Diagnosis Treatment model attempts to empower dually diagnosed individuals and to mobilize their own inner resources. Meeting patients where they are in terms of motivation serves to facilitate and strengthen their resolve, self-efficacy, and continued forward movement in improving the quality of their lives.

References

Alcoholics Anonymous: The AA Member: Medication and Other Drugs. New York, Alcoholics Anonymous World Services, 1984

American Psychiatric Association: Diagnostic and Statistical Manual of Mental Disorders, 4th Edition. Washington, DC, American Psychiatric Association, 1994

American Psychiatric Association: Practice guideline for the treatment of patients with nicotine dependence. Am J Psychiatry 153 (10, suppl):1–31, 1996

Ananth J, Vanderwater S, Kamal M, et al: Missed diagnosis of substance abuse in psychiatric patients. Hospital and Community Psychiatry 40:297–299, 1989

Andreasson S, Allebeck P, Engstrom A, et al: Cannabis and schizophrenia: a longitudinal study of Swedish conscripts. Lancet 2:1483–1486, 1987

Ballenger JC, Post RM: Kindling as a model for alcohol withdrawal syndromes. Br J Psychiatry 133:1–14, 1978

Brady K, Anton R, Ballenger JC, et al: Cocaine abuse among schizophrenic patients. Am J Psychiatry 147:1164–1167, 1990

Buckley P, Thompson P, Way L, et al: Substance abuse among patients with treatment-resistant schizophrenia: characteristics and implications for clozapine therapy. Am J Psychiatry 151:385–389, 1994

Cohen E, Henkin I: Substance abuse and lifestyle among an urban schizophrenic population: some observations. Psychiatry 58:113–120, 1995

Cuffel BJ: Prevalence estimates of substance abuse in schizophrenia and their correlates. J Nerv Ment Dis 180:589–592, 1992

DeQuardo JR, Carpenter CF, Tandon R: Patterns of substance abuse in schizophrenia: nature and significance. J Psychiatr Res 28:267–275, 1994

Dilsaver SC: The pathopsychophysiologies of substance abuse and affective disorders: an integrative model? J Clin Psychopharmacol 7:1–10, 1987

Dixon L, Haas G, Weiden PJ, et al: Acute effects of drug abuse in schizophrenic patients. Schizophr Bull 16:69–79, 1990

Drake RE, Wallach MA: Substance abuse among the mentally ill. Hospital and Community Psychiatry 40:1041–1046, 1989

Drake RE, Osher FC, Wallach MA: Alcohol use and abuse in schizophrenia: a perspective community study. J Nerv Ment Dis 177:408–414, 1989

Drake RE, Bartels SJ, Teague GB, et al: Treatment of substance abuse in severely mentally ill patients. J Nerv Ment Dis 181:606–611, 1993

Ereshefsky L: Pharmacokinetics and drug interactions: update for new antipsychotics. J Clin Psychiatry 57 (suppl 11):12–25, 1996

Ereshefsky L, Saklad SR, Watanabe MD, et al: Thiothixene pharmacokinetic interactions: a study of hepatic enzyme inducers, clearance inhibitors, and demographic variables. J Clin Psychopharmacol 11:296–300, 1991

Frederick J, Cotanch P: Self-help techniques for auditory hallucinations in schizophrenia. Issues in Mental Health Nursing 16:213–224, 1995

Gardner EL, Paredes W, Chen J: Further evidence for THC as a dopamine reuptake blocker: brain microdialysis studies. Society for Neuroscience Abstracts 16:1100, 1990

George TP, Semyak MI, Ziedonis DM, et al: Effects of clozapine on smoking in chronic schizophrenic outpatients. J Clin Psychiatry 56:344–346, 1995

George TP, Ziedonis DM, Feingold A, et al: Nicotine transdermal patch and atypical antipsychotic drugs for smoking cessation in schizophrenia. Am J Psychiatry (in press)

Glassman AH: Cigarette smoking: implications for psychiatric illness. Am J Psychiatry 150:546–553, 1993

Glazer WM, Morgenstern H: Predictors of occurrence, severity, and course of TD in an outpatient population. J Clin Psychopharmacol 8(no 4, suppl):10S–16S, 1988

Goff DC, Henderson DC, Amico BS: Cigarette smoking in schizophrenia: relationship to psychopathology and medication side effects. Am J Psychiatry 149:1189–1194, 1992

Greden JF, Procter A, Victor BS: Caffeinism associated with greater use of other psychotropic agents. Compr Psychiatry 22:565–571, 1981

Hall GH: Pharmacology of tobacco in relation to schizophrenia, in Biochemistry of Schizophrenia and Addiction: In Search of a Common Factor. Edited by Hemmings G. Baltimore, MD, Baltimore University Press, 1980, pp 199–207

Hamera E, Schneider JK, Kraenzle J, et al: Alcohol, cannabis, nicotine, and caffeine use and symptom distress in schizophrenia. J Nerv Ment Dis 183:559–565, 1995

Hellerstein DJ, Meehan B: Outpatient group therapy for schizophrenic substance abusers. Am J Psychiatry 144:1337–1339, 1987

Higgins ST, Budney AJ, Bickel WK, et al: Incentives improve outcome in outpatient behavioral treatment of cocaine dependence. Arch Gen Psychiatry 51:568–576, 1994

Janowsky DS, Davis DM: Methylphenidate, dextroamphetamine, and levamfetamine: effects on schizophrenic symptoms. Arch Gen Psychiatry 33:304–308, 1976

Kendler KS: A twin study of individuals with schizophrenia and alcoholism. Br J Psychiatry 147:48–53, 1985

Khantzian E: The self-medication hypothesis of addictive disorders: focus on heroin and cocaine dependence. Am J Psychiatry 142:1259–1264, 1985

Knudsen P, Vilmar T: Cannabis and neuroleptic agents in schizophrenia. Acta Psychiatr Scand 69:162–174, 1984

Kofoed L: Assessment of comorbid psychiatric illness and substance disorders. New Dir Ment Health Serv 50:43–55, 1991

Kofoed L, Keys A: Using group therapy to persuade dual-diagnosis patients to seek substance abuse treatment. Hospital and Community Psychiatry 39:1209–1211, 1988

Kosten TR, Nestler EJ: Clozapine attenuates cocaine conditioned place preference. Life Sci 55:PL9–PL14, 1994

Larson E: Stage II Recovery. New York, HarperCollins, 1985

Lehman H, Nair V, Kline N: Beta-endorphin and naloxone in psychiatric patients. Am J Psychiatry 136:762–766, 1979

Lysaker P, Bell M, Beam-Goulet J, et al: Relationship of positive and negative symptoms to cocaine abuse in schizophrenia. J Nerv Ment Dis 182:109–122, 1994

Markou A, Koob GF: Postcocaine anhedonia: an animal model of cocaine withdrawal. Neuropsychopharmacology 4:17–26, 1991

Mayfield D, McLeod G, Hall P: The CAGE Questionnaire: validation of a new alcoholism screening instrument. Am J Psychiatry 131:1121–1123, 1974

McCance EF, Price LH, Kosten TR, et al: Cocaethylene: pharmacology, physiology and behavioral effects in humans. J Pharmacol Exp Ther 274:215–223, 1995

McEvoy J, Freudenreich O, McGee M, et al: Clozapine decreases smoking in patients with chronic schizophrenia. Biol Psychiatry 37:550–552, 1995

Miller WR, Rollnick S: Motivational Interviewing: Preparing People to Change Addictive Behavior. New York, Guilford, 1991

Miller WR, Zweben A, DiClemente CC, et al: Motivational Enhancement Therapy Manual (DHHS Publ No ADM-92-1894). Rockville, MD, U.S. Department of Health and Human Services, 1992

Minkoff K: An integrated treatment model for dual diagnosis of psychosis and addiction. Hospital and Community Psychiatry 40:1031–1036, 1989

Mueser KT, Gingerich S: Coping With Schizophrenia. Oakland, CA, Harbinger, 1994

Mueser KT, Nishith P, Tracy JI, et al: Expectations and motives for substance use in schizophrenia. Psychiatr Clin North Am 21:367–378, 1995

Naber D, Nedopil N, Eben E: No correlation between neuroleptic-induced increase of β-endorphin serum level and therapeutic efficacy in schizophrenia. Br J Psychiatry 144:651–653, 1984

Negrete JC, Knapp WP, Douglas DE, et al: Cannabis affects the severity of schizophrenic symptoms: results of a clinical survey. Psychol Med 16:515–520, 1986

Nikkel RE: Areas of skill training for persons with mental illness and substance use disorders: building skills for successful community living. Community Ment Health J 30:61–72, 1994

Noordsy DL, Drake RE, Biesanz JC, et al: Family history of alcoholism in schizophrenia. J Nerv Ment Dis 182:651–655, 1994

Oepen G, Levy M, Saemann R, et al: A neuropsychological perspective on dual diagnosis. J Psychoactive Drugs 25:129–133, 1993

Olivera AA, Kiefer MW, Manley NK: Tardive dyskinesia in psychiatric patients with substance use disorders. Am J Drug Alcohol Abuse 16:57–66, 1990

O'Malley S, Adamse M, Heaton RK, et al: Neuropsychological impairment in chronic cocaine abusers. Am J Drug Alcohol Abuse 18:131–144, 1992

Osher FC, Kofoed LL: Treatment of patients with psychiatric and psychoactive substance abuse disorders. Hospital and Community Psychiatry 40:1025–1030, 1989

Prochaska JO, DiClemente CC, Norcross JC: In search of how people change: applications to addictive disorders. Am Psychol 47:1102–1114, 1992

Project MATCH Research Group: Matching alcoholism treatments to client heterogeneity: treatment main effects and matching effects on drinking during treatment. J Stud Alcohol 59:631–639, 1998

Rao S, Ziedonis DM, Kosten TR: The pharmacotherapy for cocaine dependence. Psychiatric Annals 25:363–368, 1995

Regier DA, Farmer ME, Rae DS, et al: Comorbidity of mental disorders with alcohol and other drug abuses. JAMA 264:2511–2518, 1990

Sandyk R: Cigarette smoking: effects on cognitive functions and drug-induced parkinsonism in chronic schizophrenia. Int J Neurosci 70:193–197, 1993

Satel JA, Lieberman JA: Schizophrenia and substance abuse. Psychiatr Clin North Am 16:401–412, 1991

Schneier FR, Siris SG: A review of psychoactive substance use and abuse in schizophrenia: patterns of drug choice. J Nerv Ment Dis 175:641–652, 1987

Seibyl JP, Satel SL, Anthony D, et al: Effects of cocaine on hospital course in schizophrenia. J Nerv Ment Dis 181:31–37, 1993

Seltzer ML: The Michigan Alcoholism Screening Test: the quest for a new diagnostic instrument. Am J Psychiatry 127:89–94, 1971

Serper MR, Alpert M, Richardson NA, et al: Clinical effects of recent cocaine use on patients with acute schizophrenia. Am J Psychiatry 152:1464–1469, 1995

Sevy S, Kay SR, Opler LA, et al: Significance of cocaine history in schizophrenia. J Nerv Ment Dis 178:642–648, 1990

Shaner A, Khalsa E, Roberts L, et al: Unrecognized cocaine use among schizophrenic patients. Am J Psychiatry 150:758–762, 1993

Stahl SM: Essential Psychopharmacology. New York, Cambridge University Press, 1996

Strakowski SM, Tohen M, Flaum M, et al: Substance abuse in psychotic disorders: associations with affective syndromes. Schizophr Res 14:73–81, 1994

Test MA, Wallisch LS, Allness DJ, et al: Substance use in young adults with schizophrenic disorders. Schizophr Bull 15:465–476, 1989

Tracy JI, Josiassen RC, Bellack AS: Neuropsychology of dual diagnosis: understanding the combined effects of schizophrenia and substance use disorders. Clin Psychol Rev 15:67–97, 1995

Vanover KE, Piercey MF, Woolverton WL: Evaluation of the reinforcing and discriminative stimulus effects of cocaine in combination with (+)-AJ76 or clozapine. J Pharmacol Exp Ther 266:780–789, 1993

Westermeyer JW: Schizophrenia and drug abuse, in American Psychiatric Press Review of Psychiatry, Vol 11. Edited by Tasman A, Riba MB. Washington, DC, American Psychiatric Press, 1992, pp 379–401

Zaretsky A, Rector NA, Seeman MV, et al: Current cannabis use and tardive dyskinesia. Schizophr Res 11:3–8, 1993

Ziedonis DM: Comorbid psychopathology and cocaine addiction, in Clinician's Guide to Cocaine Addiction. Edited by Kosten TR, Kleber HD. New York, Guilford, 1992, pp 337–360

Ziedonis DM: Substance abuse prevention strategies for psychiatric patients, in Handbook on Drug Abuse Prevention: A Comprehensive Strategy to Prevent the Abuse of Alcohol and Other Drugs. Edited by Coombs RH, Ziedonis DM. Boston, MA, Allyn & Bacon, 1995, pp 445–469

Ziedonis DM, Fisher W: Assessment and treatment of comorbid substance abuse in individuals with schizophrenia. Psychiatric Annals 24:477–483, 1994

Ziedonis DM, Fisher W: Motivation based assessment and treatment of substance abuse in patients with schizophrenia. New Directions in Psychiatry 16:1-8, 1996

Ziedonis DM, George TP: Schizophrenia and nicotine use: report of a pilot smoking cessation program and review of neurobiological and clinical issues. Schizophr Bull 23:247–254, 1997

Ziedonis DM, Kosten TR: Pharmacotherapy improves treatment outcome in depressed cocaine addicts. J Psychoactive Drugs 23:417–425, 1991

Ziedonis DM, Trudeau K: Motivation to quit using substances among individuals with schizophrenia: implications for a motivation-based treatment model. Schizophr Bull 23:229–238, 1997

Ziedonis DM, Richardson T, Lee E, et al: Adjunctive desipramine in the treatment of cocaine abusing schizophrenics. Psychopharmacol Bull 28:309–314, 1992

Ziedonis DM, Kosten TR, Glazer WM, et al: Nicotine dependence and schizophrenia. Hospital and Community Psychiatry 45:204–206, 1994

Ziedonis D, Williams J, Corrigan P, et al: Management of schizophrenia and substance abuse. Psychiatric Annals 30:67–75, 2000

Zisook S, Heaton R, Moranville J, et al: Past substance abuse and clinical course of schizophrenia. Am J Psychiatry 149:552–553, 1992

Index

*Page numbers printed in **boldface** type refer to tables or figures.*